WP 17 WIL

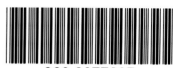

369 0077297

date shown below.

Circumareolar Techniques
for Breast Surgery

Tolbert S. Wilkinson   Adrien E. Aiache   Luiz S. Toledo

Circumareolar Techniques for Breast Surgery

WITH 149 ILLUSTRATIONS IN 376 PARTS

Springer-Verlag

New York   Berlin   Heidelberg   London   Paris
Tokyo   Hong Kong   Barcelona   Budapest

Tolbert S. Wilkinson, M.D., F.A.C.S.
The Institute for Aesthetic Plastic Surgery
One Oak Hills Place
1901 Babcock, Suite 200
San Antonio, TX 78229
USA

Adrien E. Aiache, M.D.
9884 Little Santa Monica Blvd.
Beverly Hills, CA 90212
USA

Luiz S. Toledo, M.D.
Clinica Toledo
Rupublica do Libano 904
São Paulo, SP 04502-001
Brazil

Library of Congress Cataloging-in-Publication Data
Wilkinson, Tolbert S., 1937–
Circumareolar techniques for breast surgery / Tolbert S.
Wilkinson, Adrien E. Aiache, Luiz S. Toledo.
p. cm.
Includes bibliographical references and index.
ISBN 0-387-94378-1
1. Mammaplasty. 2. Mammaplasty—Complications—Prevention.
I. Aiache, Adrien E. II. Toledo, Luiz Sérgio. III. Title.
[DNLM: 1. Breast—surgery. 2. Mammaplasty—methods. WP 910
W687c 1995]
RD539.8.W54, 1995
618.1'9059—dc20
DNLM/DLC
for Library of Congress   94-32696

Printed on acid-free paper.

Production coordinated by Publishing Network and managed by Laura Carlson;
manufacturing supervised by Jacqui Ashri.
Typeset by ATLIS Graphics, Mechanicsburg, PA.
Printed and bound by Maple-Vail, York, PA.
Printed in the United States of America.

9 8 7 6 5 4 3 2 1

ISBN 0-387-94378-1 Springer-Verlag   New York   Berlin   Heidelberg

Dedication and Acknowledgments

Our interest in the circumareolar technique of breast surgery began in our respective practices and culminated in the exchange of ideas and techniques that produced this book and improved our results with the various aspects of this technique dependent of breast surgery. Despite our different backgrounds and practices in different locales, we have encountered the same problems in our patients, to whom we dedicate this work. We also dedicate this volume to our respective teachers—mine include Drs. Kenneth Pickrell, Nicholas Georgiade, and Francis X. Paletta, from whom I received my training in the basis of plastic surgery. We too strive for excellence, but retain a pragmatic evaluation of our efforts. In their footsteps, we constantly strive to improve the technical and emotional aspects of breast surgery.

We thank our wives for their support and uniquely feminine viewpoints on this aspect of our endeavors. The exchange of ideas that constantly occurs in plastic surgery has benefitted the three of us as well as those who have led the way in similar surgical explorations. We give particular thanks to Drs. Ulrich Hinderer, Paul McKissock, and Louis Benelli. Each of these men had the foresight and the personal bravery to develop new operative procedures in a most unforgiving area of the female body, and to blaze pathways for those of us who have followed and elaborated upon their techniques and their insights. We also extend our debt of gratitude to the American Society for Aesthetic Plastic Surgery, the International Review of Aesthetic Plastic Surgery organization, and members of these societies who have influenced our careers: Richard Stark and John Lewis. Also, our thanks to other current pioneers: Drs. Larry Schlesinger,

Melvyn Dinner, Mine Kurtay, and especially Scott Spear, whose practical reasoned approach to the problems of breast hypertrophy and descent has influenced us to evaluate each new procedure with his same attention to detail and comparative evaluation. Without the help and encouragement of Ms. Esther Gumpert of Springer-Verlag, my staff, and my wife, Suzanne, there would be no manuscript, photographs, or patient histories that comprise this volume. And, finally, I am grateful to my polo teammates, who put up with my time constraints!

T.S.W.

This book has been written in collaboration with Drs. Wilkinson and Toledo in order to assemble our diverse experiences in the accomplishment of the technique. The technique, which is old, has been revised by Dr. Benelli; and since we were interested and courses were given along these lines at the American Society of Plastic and Reconstructive Surgery meeting, it was felt that a textbook would be useful.

I want to thank Drs. Wilkinson and Toledo for their excellent contribution, as well as my family, my wife, and my staff, who have been very helpful in allowing me to take this task to completion. We want to thank the American Society for Aesthetic Plastic Surgery for allowing us to give the course concerning this technique, as well as Drs. Benelli and Hinderer, who have been helpful in giving their advice as well as imparting their knowledge on the history of this technique.

A.E.A.

My experience with the periareolar technique during the 1970s was not a happy one. Although I did not perform the technique myself, it was based on viewing the postoperative results that came to my office or were presented in congresses. The idea did not grow on me.

In 1985, an article in a glossy woman's magazine showed the impressive pre- and postoperative results of Dr. Ricardo Bustos with only one incision around the areola. In Brazil, where the inverted T technique was evolved and refined, it was difficult to think of a different approach to breast reduction. This periareolar technique was the procedure many of our patients were waiting for, and they started asking for it.

My first patient wanting this technique insisted that I find a way to perform the periareolar reduction. I had to develop my own approach to this operation, and the results were good. Patients like her are hard to come by, and I thank her for the support I needed to perform my first case.

I would like to thank Dr. William E.P. Callia, from whom I learnt not only about aesthetic plastic surgery, but also how to recognize a real advance in our field.

Dr. Ruy Raia, my professor of reconstructive surgery, a man who knows how to delegate responsibility, gave me the opportunity for vast hands-on experience.

I am grateful to Esther Gumpert, our editor at Springer-Verlag.

I thank my parents, Pedro and Yvonne, for their unwavering support; and my son, Juliano, and my daughters, Isabella and Valentina, who have had to put up with my absence, although they are always on my mind.

I also thank my wife, Kate, who is dedicated not only to our family, but also to everything that involves my professional life; she is the rudder that keeps us in pleasant waters.

L.S.T.

Contents

Introduction

The genesis of this book was the enthusiastic response to a teaching course organized by Dr. Tolbert Wilkinson and presented by the three authors of this text at the 1992 American Society for Plastic and Reconstructive Surgeons annual meeting. Because we had so often borrowed ideas and expertise from each other, and yet pursued our individual goals and techniques, it was appropriate to prepare a text that would encompass all of the techniques as well as the extensive experience of the authors. Although the operation is still in transition, experience with the procedure definitely improves the cosmetic results. We offer a series of technical changes that may be adapted and improved by the experienced plastic surgeon for the benefit of the patients.

The Circumareolar Procedures

Tolbert S. Wilkinson

Like most American surgeons, my interest in the circumareolar technique was stimulated by the presentation and then publication on a new mastopexy operation by Roger Bartels.[1] Bartels quoted studies that showed that horizontal and vertical breast scars in 1976 averaged 18 mm in width in the vertical direction and 8 to 9 mm in width laterally, regardless of the technique or type of closure. He commented that patients submitting to mastopexy were trading ptosis for extensive and perhaps unacceptable scars. Even in 1994, we have problems with all scars, but more so in the horizontal direction. Bartel's comments certainly struck a chord in me. In his original paper, the mastopexies described were performed on very small breasts. Nevertheless, areolae increased in size dramatically. Many of his cases were patients that we would treat by breast augmentation today, with acceptable tiny incisions. Others would be candidates for the modern circumareolar technique.

Another article, by Barry Davidson,[2] described the use of the circumareolar technique for gynecomastia—certainly a smaller degree of ptosis. By removing only soft tissue, there was little reason to expect areolar stretch and indeed none oc-

curred, as can be seen in the photographs in that article. I had used the circle technique in 1976 in several small mastopexies but was concerned because the areolar scars seemed no less obvious than the mastopexy areolar scars (Figure 1.1) generated using other techniques, and it was certainly a more difficult procedure. Nevertheless, these early patients quickly expressed their satisfaction with the single scar and with avoiding chest scars (Figure 1.2). But times and customs change: in 1976 few women wore revealing clothing; scar visibility is more important to patients today.

The infolding technique for small mastopexies (described in Chapter 7) first came to our attention with the presentation and later publication from the Baylor College of Medicine (Houston, TX) by Onur Erol and Melvin Spira.[3] Now we were really interested. Cases were shown with a complete circle excision for exposure and areolar lift. Erol chose cases requiring little skin excision and the lifted breasts were quite small by today's standard. This left the rest of us to deal with the larger mastopexy on our own! Discussions of surgery to correct a concentric excision for the areolar breast ("Snoopy" deformity) included cir-

Major Additions Since Erol's First Cases (1976)
1. Deepithelialized ring
2. Liposuction
3. Resetting of inframammary fold
4. Creation of cone shape
5. Double "Benelli" suture
6. Toledo triangle/Texas diamond

cle excisions as well. Many surgeons saw the complications of the "doughnut" mastopexy and dismissed it entirely.

In the next 5 years the procedure changed very little. Surgeons still employed multiple subcutaneous sutures of a delayed dissolving type, such as Vicryl or Dexon, and surface half-buried mattress sutures of Nylon, the same procedure that is used today in the standard reduction mammo-

plasty. Unfortunately, the scars generated by this technique did not smooth as quickly as possible. In patient J.V. (Figure 1.3A–D) breast shape was maintained by the addition of small breast prostheses and the areolae did not expand, but the irregularity of the areolae and the inevitable stretch made the procedure less satisfactory. The other situation, called "star gazing" (upward areolar position change) occurred less frequently, as illustrated by patient J.V. (Figure 1.4). After a period of 5 years there was continued stretch of the lower quadrant of the breasts, leaving the nipples at a higher position in relation to the overall shape. This is the reason why many of the subsequent nipple positionings performed on patients between 1985 and 1990 involved the choice of a lower nipple-areolar spot, because of our fear of star gazing. "Star gazing" is a phenomenon of breast descent, commonly seen in breast

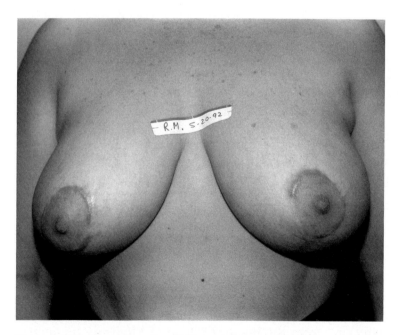

Figure 1.1. Choosing the lollipop skin excision to complement a circumareolar-type lift is no guarantee against complications, as illustrated by patient R.M., seen 1 year following a mastopexy performed by a very good surgeon in our area and referred to us for aftercare. She has continued to wear brassieres and has used the recommended oils to massage her scar areas faithfully. Nevertheless, at the end of 1 year scar hypertrophy is noted, as is further descent of the breast, despite the effect of the "skin brassiere." Notice also the extreme widening of the lollipop incision between each areola and the inframammary fold. This reemphasizes the fact that a skin excision does not add to the longevity of a mastopexy or reduction. Good internal repair and multilayered cross-over suturing are far more important that the effect of the skin and, as shown in this case, we would have only one area of scar hypertrophy to deal with rather than those illustrated.

Figure 1.2. (A) Appearance of patient B.S. in 1979, at the time she underwent circumareolar mastopexy. (B) Patient B.S. in 1990, years after the circumareolar mastopexy. There has been some descent of the breast, as expected, but no more than in my other patients who underwent mastopexy by a variety of other methods. Although she was not concerned, the widening of the scars was an area for improvement. Notice that the areolae did not expand.

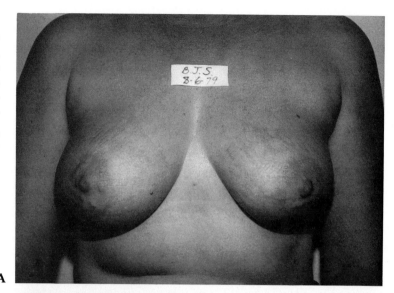

A

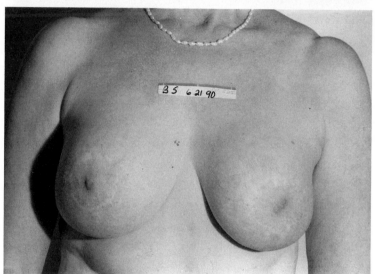

B

reduction patients, in which the nipple has been placed at the upper limits of normal (Figure 1.5). Subsequent refinements in circumareolar surgery have been directed toward the prevention of this problem and have been largely successful. With individual variations that occur in the female population, it is unrealistic to expect that all patients will resist the effects of gravity on nipple position and contour of the lower breast.

The scar itself, as produced by the circumareolar procedure, is no more predictable or controllable than the circumareolar scar generated by standard mastopexies or reduction. However,

although the major concern for many patients is clothing choices, the newer technique eliminates irritation of the horizontal scar by brassieres, reduces the probability of loss of sensation, and most of all minimizes the visible reminders of the prior abnormality.

As noted, our initial experience with the circumareolar technique was not good. The circumareolar scars required frequent revisions (although currently no more so than the circumareolar scar of our standard mastopexy reduction). Early results included flattening of the breast, fullness above the areola, areolar descent to the center of

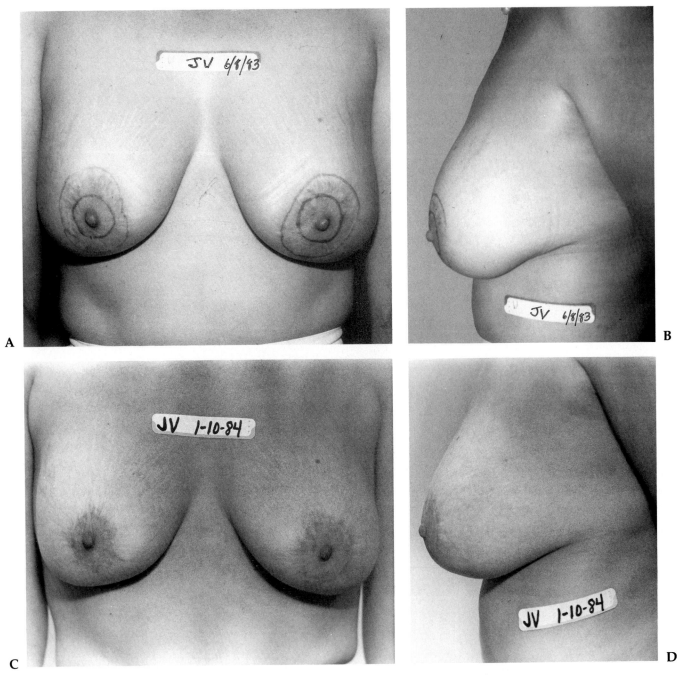

Figure 1.3. In 1984, before the adoption of the deepithelialized circle and the circular advancing sutures of Benelli, irregular periareolar scarring occurred with some frequency as shown in patient J.V. (**A** and **B**). Whether due to the inherent problems of the ptotic breast or to the surgical technique, revisions are carried out in this group of patients with some frequency. My initial impression, however, was that revisions were required no less frequently in the circumareolar patients than in those in which standard mastopexies had been performed with augmentation mammoplasty prostheses. Notice in the prerevision photograph (**C**) that the weight of the prostheses has stretched the lower portions of the breasts, causing the nipple-areolar complexes to ride upward. In large breast reduction this complication is called "star gazing."

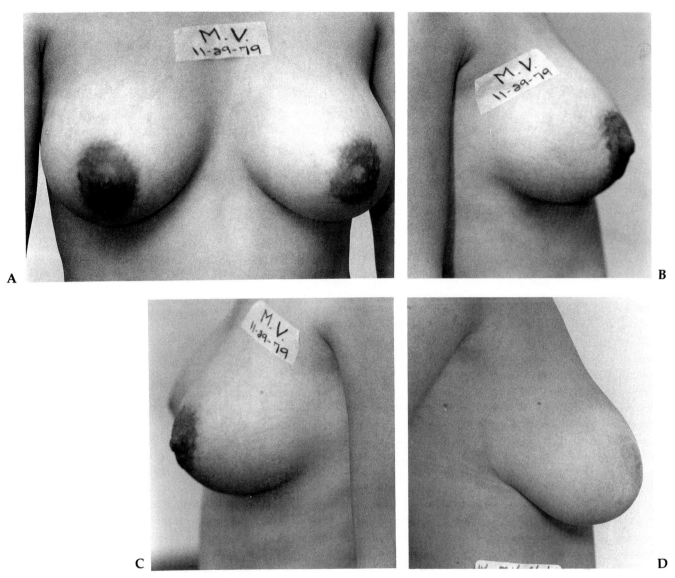

Figure 1.4. Breast descent occurs in many mastopexy patients, as shown in **(A)** through **(F)**. Patient M.V. underwent an augmentation of moderately ptotic breasts in 1979. We were not as strict then in our insistence on brassiere support, and stretching occurred to a greater degree than desired in this patient, as shown in **(D)**. A circumareolar mastopexy was required in 1984, and is shown in **(E)** and **(F)**, taken 7 months postoperatively. The internal overlapping repair with areolar repositioning appears to be holding quite well. This category of patient is difficult for several reasons. Without good internal tissue support, all mastopexies will require revisions. The procedure, discussed in Chapter 7, of doubly reinforcing the lower half of these ptotic breasts has certainly delayed the inevitable descent, but is not preventive in all cases.

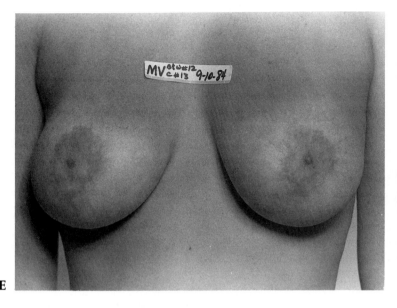

E

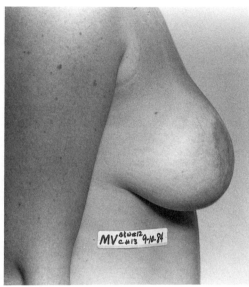

F

Figure 1.4. *Continued*

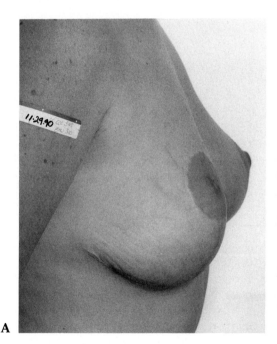

A

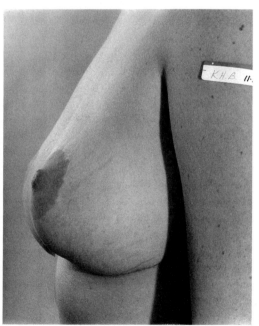

B

Figure 1.5. Multiple revision for "star gazing." A further stimulus for the development of circumareolar techniques was incurred by patients such as this lady, in which the areolae are too high and revisions have not effected an acceptable shape. "Star gazing" is the description given to such a breast reduction patient. Her complaint was that her nipples appeared above her brassiere while her scar extended below her brassiere! Her breasts were also quite flat and misshapen (**A–C**). The first phase of the correction involved closing the areolar site to reposition the nipples at a lower spot, and adding textured breast prostheses for fullness. Two years postoperatively, scar hypertrophy was still present and full expansion of the left side had not been affected (**D** and **E**). The next revision, in March 1992, included advancement of the skin over the scar beds, revision of the areolar scars, a third revision of the lateral and medial horizontal limb scars, and a repositioning of the prosthesis on the left for symmetry. Shape and symmetry have been achieved (**F**). Unfortunately, breast reductions requiring multiple revisions to a greater or lesser degree are not uncommon. With the circumareolar technique, there is less likelihood of such occurrences.

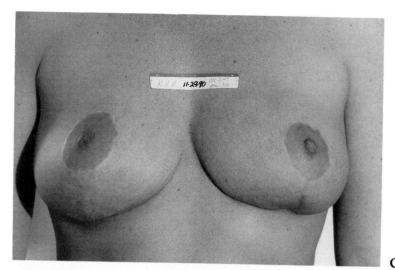

C

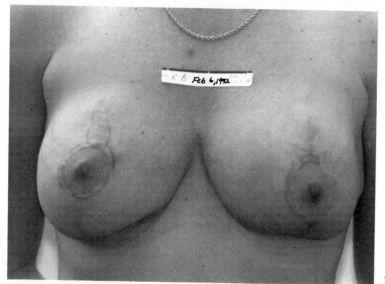

D

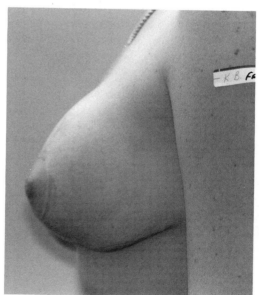

E

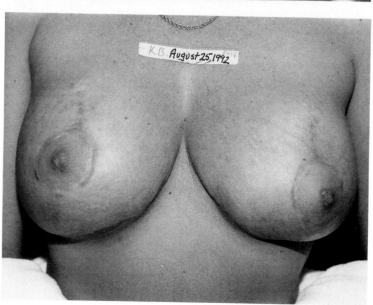

F

the circle, and, most disturbingly, areolar stretch with concomitant scar hypertrophy. These complications made the procedure less desirable.

Thanks to authors who had contributed technical innovations in the 1970s, there was some enthusiasm for the procedure. More recent publications in the literature, however, must be considered as setbacks. Photographs still show a flat "pancake" breast with huge areolae. This is no longer an acceptable "trade-off" for avoiding vertical or horizontal scars! With increasing familiarity with the procedure, and the incorporation of the newer technical maneuvers described in this book, the circumareolar technique has become quite satisfactory to physician and patient, even though there are limitations and imperfections.

The circumareolar technique has become increasingly popular in South America and in Europe. The techniques of infolding through a small incision gave an elevation to small breasts with only a short incision at the areolar edge. When the areola needed elevation, a small excision of circumareolar skin was incorporated to reposition the nipple-areolar complex upward. With success in the smaller breast lifts and reductions, measures were adopted to prevent distortion if a mammary prosthesis was added for augmentation. In the small and large mastopexy, these measures eliminated areolar stretch. Soon the procedure was extended to larger and larger breast reductions.

With the aggressive use of liposuction, it has become apparent that the currently popular "lollipop" vertical skin excision is rarely required. We had often used liposuction for final adjustments of the breast volume in reduction surgery, but the aggressive use of liposuction as a primary tool soon became an invaluable part of the circumareolar approach. Liposuction alone has been employed as a primary procedure for certain categories of individuals who do not require the elegance of breast reshaping along with mass reduction, a further indication of the value of this technique in circumareolar reduction mammoplasty.

And what about small, or even large, breast reduction? Could these patients reap the benefit

> *Breast Reduction*
> Superior pedicle—Benelli
> Subcutaneous Pitanguy—Wilkinson et al.
> With liposuction—Toledo

of the circumareolar technique, if we, the surgeons, could solve the technical problems?

Once the concept of creating a complete breast shape subcutaneously was grasped, the search was underway for techniques to ensure that the round, elevated mound was of long duration, and for methods to reduce the scarring around the areola and the spreading of the areolar diameter. These techniques and improvements have come from a number of sources.

As can be seen in these pages, we have progressed from the initial attempt to create a multi-layered closure with buried and superficial sutures to a concept of tension-relaxing sutures placed at a distance from the areolar edge. The preference of the authors of this textbook is for the circumareolar suture, popularized by Louis Benelli. Other authors, such as Larry Schleslinger, use criss-crossing sutures, which achieve the same relief of tension. The basic principle is to avoid any tension where the edges of the breast skin meet the edges of the reduced areola. The addition of liposuction for sculpturing is an important adjunct.

Madeleine Lejour addressed the question of breast reduction by liposuction alone, in her discussion of Eugene Courtiss's series,[4] by emphasizing that tissue resection is an essential part of any breast reduction. "The degree of ptosis left by liposuction alone would be considered unpleasant by my patients." As Dr. Lejour writes, such patients complained their breasts were "jumping out of their bras" when they would lean forward and falling laterally when they would lie in a bed, and they would "regularly beg for firm and high breasts."

This is the purpose of this text: to familiarize knowledgeable plastic surgeons with the techniques of using liposuction, along with resection, to create firm, high breasts without any more scarring than is absolutely necessary.

I certainly agree with Lejour's statement that "we surgeons tend to accept the scars that the patients do not," and that it would be marvelous if patients could improve the shape of their breasts after the volume changes of pregnancy and lactation without tissue removal, but this unfortunately is not the case. Leaving aside the question of liposuction aspirates that might encounter small malignancies that could not be traced to a specific area of the breast, the fact is that breast skin will retract only to a certain degree. In my opinion, the "skin brassiere" procedure is helpful but is not as important as the coning of the breast tissue. This coning in the reduction patient requires removal of tissue. The techniques that we employ for mastopexy involve repositioning of tissue, and in breast repair, reinforcing breast tissue. All involve the principles of "circumareolar mastopexy," which is detailed in the following chapters. I have called on two experts in circumareolar mastopexy to add their discussions in specific areas.

> Patients detest horizontal scars
> Surgeons have to deal with only one scar
> It's not that hard to do!

Adrien Aiache and Luiz S. Toledo have been leaders in the adoption of new ideas into practical working plastic surgery procedures. I trust you will enjoy the variations that they present and the modifications that differ from my own. Even though there may be some repetition, repetition by itself is not a disadvantage when one is evaluating a new procedure.

Readers should propose the following questions:

1. "Will it work for me, and how difficult will it be?"
2. "Is the advantage of minimizing scarring worth the disadvantage of the slow resolution of the periareolar scar, and any uncertainties regarding long-term effects?"

Readers will also note that many preliminary cases are shown; this has been done for several reasons. We demonstrate the problems encountered between 1976 and 1986, and the improvements that were well developed by 1990. This limits the long-term follow-up for many of the patients. In addition, it is important that one become familiar with the appearance of the breast in the early relaxation phase and be prepared for the differences in appearance that resolve with time.

In summary, circumareolar mastopexy reduction and repair is a "hands-on" experience perfectly suited to innovative plastic surgeons who can make decisions in the operating room and can modify a procedure for their own skills and their patients' needs. This operation is still in transition, as are many of our procedures. At this point, it may be safely stated that the complication rate is equal to or less than that of standard reduction procedures of all types, and the same applies to mastopexy. With increasing familiarity, the circumareolar procedure will become as comfortable and as predictable for each individual surgeon as it has become for the three of us.

Advantages of the Circumareolar Approach

There are two additional advantages to the circumareolar approach for mastopexy or reduction. The first is the enhanced access to the interior of the breast for palpation and possible biopsy, and a more efficient expansion and break-up of the fibrocystic component. Because the incidence of breast cancer is neither increased nor decreased in patients with mastopexy, reduction, or breast implants, the addition of a breast prosthesis for creation of the fullness preferred by most American mastopexy candidates is in this respect an additional plus, because the patient can do a more efficient self-examination: small breast lesions are more easily palpated with the fingertip technique in implant patients than in those without implants. In fact, a certain degree of capsular contracture makes breast examination easier. Complete capsular contracture, on the other hand, has the opposite effect. We instruct our patients with soft breasts to use the two-hand technique, as shown in Figure 1.6A and B. The patient shown in Figure 1.6C is typical of several young women who literally saved their own lives by having breast prostheses added during crescent mastopexy.

The second advantage to placement of a prosthesis during mastopexy of the circumareolar or crescent type is that this central incision allows one free access for physical expansion (Figure 1.6D). I believe that physical expansion of the breast parenchyma by digital pressure is more efficient and helpful than by the use of a temporary expander. With the prosthesis in place, one can easily press upward and outward in various directions until the inherent tuberous ligaments and bands of fibrous reaction give way. The result is a softer breast with more space for the prosthesis.

Figure 1.6. One advantage of adding a breast prosthesis rather than infolding is the obvious fullness and contour that are preferred by North American women. A second advantage is the ease of self-examination. Although it is well known that the presence of a breast prosthesis does not increase the incidence of breast cancer, it does not decrease it either. Small tumors are pushed upward by the prosthesis and are consequently more easily detected at a smaller size by finger tip palpation. In the technique illustrated, the patient is being shown how to examine the posterior surface of the breast: **(A)** with one hand in position above the areola, the finger tips of the other hand are curved upward and **(B)** the implant is displaced. A stroking maneuver will detect new growths. Patients may prefer to do this with two hands as illustrated or with the finger and thumb. Three of my patients have detected malignant growths on the undersurface of the breast that were not detected on multiple-view mammograms. **(C)** In this patient, a small nodule was pushed upward by her breast implant. She had undergone an areolar elevation (our type C-II) many years previously and detected the mass with her usual finger tip and two-hand self-examination. Once we confirmed it, we gave her a 30-day trial of vitamin E. Many such masses will disappear, because the majority are tiny cysts. In her case, it did not and subsequent biopsy revealed this to be a very early intraductal carcinoma. **(D)** The same patient, 4 months later, after she had undergone a simple excision of the area from within, with internal rotation of capsule flaps, and a series of radiation treatments. Our oncologist assured me that her cure rate is extremely high because of the early detection. Had she not had the prosthesis, the mass would have been undetectable for months or even years, and would not have been as easily controlled.

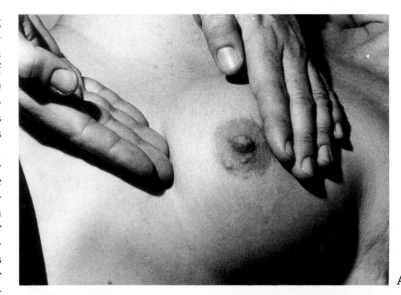

A

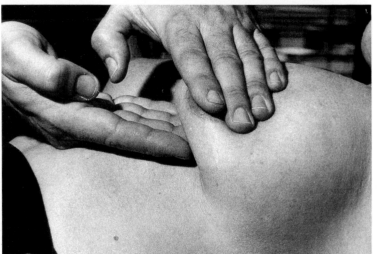

B

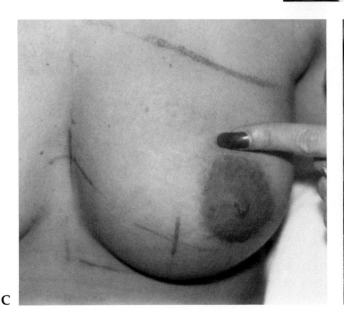

C

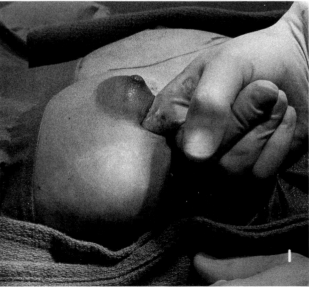

D

Ptosis: Classification and Choice of Procedures

I proposed a classification for breast augmentation candidates that was published in 1978,[6] 1983,[7] and 1989[8]; the classification system was designed to indicate which patients suffered ptosis as an effect of the ageing process in subsequent years, and what should be offered: simple breast augmentation versus the lifting of the areola, or mastopexy. No mention was made of the circumareolar technique in this earlier text.

For the purpose of this book, we call the tight, fibrotic, and unexpanded breast augmentation patient type A. Today, we use textured prostheses and rely on internal manual stretching to expand a capsule. The use of textured prostheses has dramatically reduced the contracture rate.

Breast contracture is not often seen in my practice in the type B patient, in which there is little ptosis, but some postpartum stretching may be seen. This is the ideal patient. Internal stretching is still important to maintain lateral and medial expansion, but type B patients, unlike type C patients, are not cautioned zealously regarding the necessity of the wearing of brassieres. Our type C patients fall into the ptosis group that for the purposes of this book are subdivided into categories C-1, C-2, C-3, and C-4.

Categories C-1 and C-2

In category C-1 are those women with mild to moderate ptosis and atrophy of breast tissue. Restoration of fullness is the major objective. A 1.5- to 2-cm inferior periareolar junction incision allows a repositioning of the inframammary fold from within, and textured breast prosthetic augmentation (Figure 1.7). The repositioning of the fold aids in concealing the breast descent and the areola is pushed upward.

If moderate ptosis is accompanied by atrophy of the breasts, the first alternative to standard mastopexy may be proposed for approval. Rather than totally reshaping the breast with obligatory external scarring as in standard mastopexy de-

Personal Contraindications
1. Long breasts
2. Impatient patient
3. Poor skin quality
4. Age
5. Reduction patient who wishes to be small

Figure 1.7. *Left:* Schematic of the moderate breast ptosis of the type C-1 patient. *Right:* Treatment by repositioning of the inframammary fold from within, and textured breast prosthetic augmentation, restores fullness.

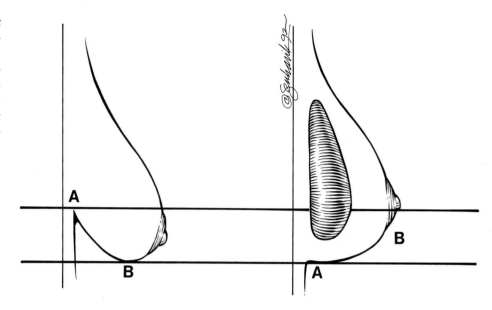

signs, we illustrate a compromise. An illusion of mastopexy correction is created by prosthetic augmentation and lowering of the inframammary fold (Figure 1.8A–D) from within.

Technical aspects of category C-1 correction are as follows: a curvilinear incision along the junction of areola and breast skin in the lower third of the areolar circumference is sufficient for development of a submammary pocket. Later, subcuticular closure of this incision rarely leaves a detectable scar. Medial and superior sharp scissor dissection allows a choice of a wide-based, low-profile textured prosthesis of a size consistent with the patient's wishes for superior fullness and cleavage without excessive forward protrusion. Under direct vision, scissor dissection inferiorly lowers the position of the inframammary fold 1 to 2 cm. A solution of local anesthetic (bupivacaine [Marcaine]) with epinephrine, a cephalosporin C analog antibiotic (cefazolin [Kefzol], 500 mg/side), and a glucocorticoid (methylprednizolone [Solu-Medrol], 20 mg/side) is instilled by a removable catheter during closure.

More than 200 such patients were reevaluated after 2 to 5 years. Continued ptosis occurred in less than 10%. In only five had the degree of ptosis progressed to an extent requiring mastopexy for correction.

As shown in Figures 1.8 through 1.10, the C-2 patients achieve a longer lasting and more natural result by surgical elevation of the areola. This procedure was nicely described as a "crescent mastopexy" by Charles Puckett et al. in 1985.[9] Lowering of the inframammary fold is usually a useful component if it is not overdone (Figure 1.11). Excessive lowering of the inframammary fold will predispose to the deformity discussed in Chapter 10 on breast repair.

The crescent mastopexy, combined with a large breast prosthesis, often gives the exact self-image desired by the patient. In contrast to South American patients, the women of Texas generally prefer fullness and, of course, do not care for the "trade-off" scar of standard mastopexy because of clothing styles. The degree of ptosis presented by patient J.C. in 1988 (Figure 1.9A–C) is typical of the majority of mastopexy series reported from other areas in the plastic surgery literature. Our patients are offered the choice of mastopexy (if they are content with a smaller B-cup shape), or crescent lift, which we have described as type C-2. Excising the ellipse of soft tissue above the areola allows for its repositioning. This patient is again shown, 5 years later, in Figure 1.9D–F. By wearing brassieres and caring for her skin, and by maintaining a healthful lifestyle, she has experienced no further descent of the breasts. The contour is perfectly acceptable and the scars have faded to a minimum. Each such patient is advised, as a further incentive to continue wearing

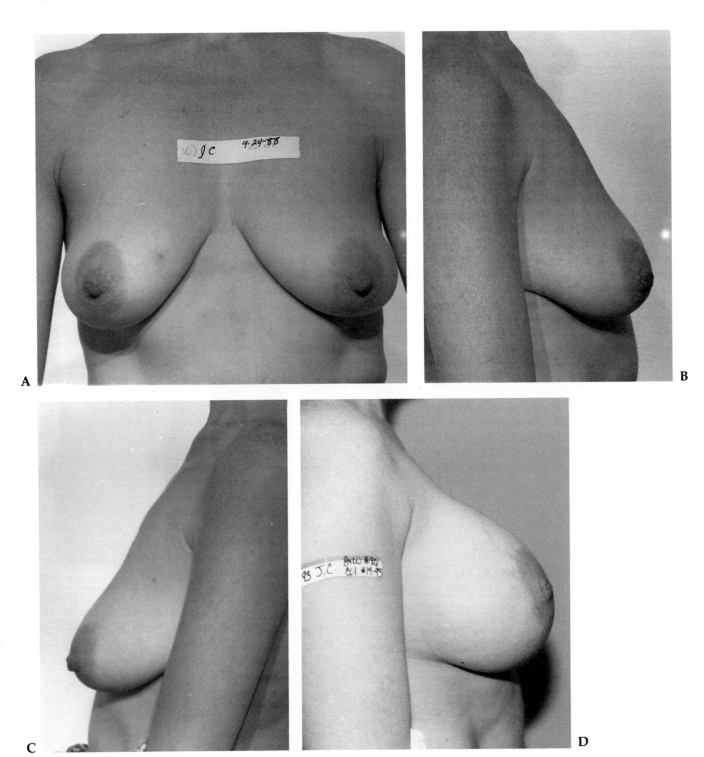

Figure 1.8. Treatment of J.C., a patient with type C-1 ptosis with atrophy. **(A–C)** Before treatment. **(D–F)** After treatment by repositioning of the inframammary fold and prosthetic augmentation: an illusion of mastopexy has been achieved, without external scarring.

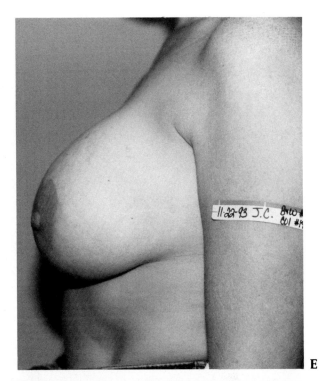

E

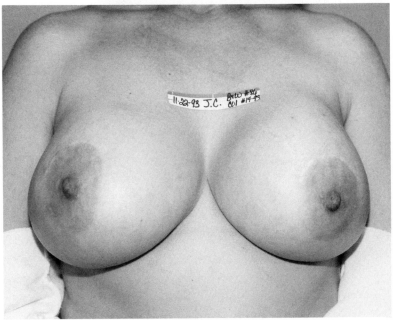

F

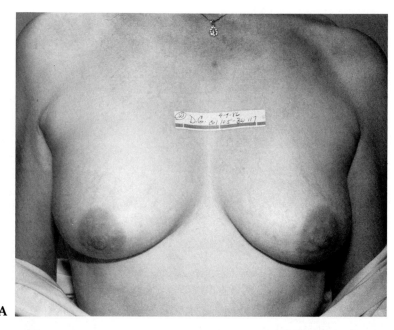

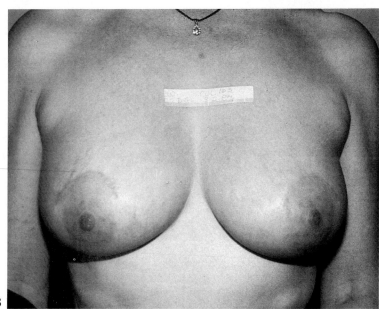

Figure 1.9. Another example of type C-1 correction by "crescent mastopexy." **(A, C)** Before treatment; **(B, D)** after treatment.

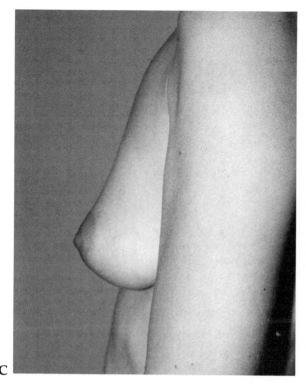

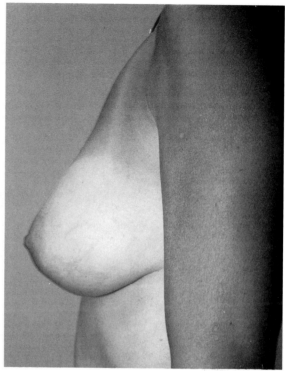

C

D

breast support, that it is far easier to control the appearance of the half-circle scar than the full-circle scar generated by mastopexy. It is likely that these patients will have some type of further lifting or internal repair, or even a full circumareolar lift, in the future, but patient J.C. illustrates the common experience in our clinic: these patients are well motivated and few of our type C ptotic breast patients have required mastopexy in the 15 years during which this alternative procedure has been widely employed.

Category C-3—Post-Prosthesis Ptosis

A number of augmentation patients develop localized stretching of the breast (discussed in more detail in Chapter 10) with or without descent of the nipple areolar complex. I call this group C-3. Because these patients often have a tiny partial-circle periareolar incision, which is for all practical purposes invisible, and because scars outside of the areolar-skin junction are unpredictable, the

techniques of circumareolar reinforcement and repair are applied in this group as well. The main difference is that the incision is short and the internal repair is more difficult, owing to the more limited visualization. In Chapter 10 we deal with patients who wish to have their breast prostheses removed. A larger incision is required, as is a wider subcutaneous dissection, to allow recontouring of the infolding breast tissue mound. If a breast prosthesis is replaced, the left-to-right overfolding gives greater support to the lower half of the breast, and resetting the inframammary fold to a higher position and shortening the stretched tissue length between the areola and inframammary fold elevate the nipple-areolar complex. Many of these patients request larger prostheses because of the atrophy effects and lateral gravitational drift induced by pregnancy. Others have experienced breast descent due to pressure from an overlying pectoralis muscle. In my practice, I rarely place prostheses under the muscle for this reason. The new textured prostheses induce less contracture and, therefore, I make every effort to avoid submuscular place-

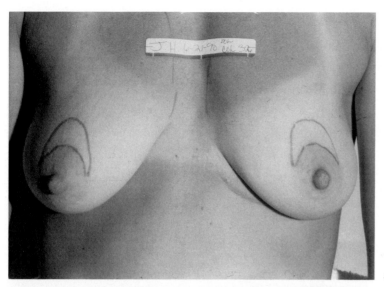

A

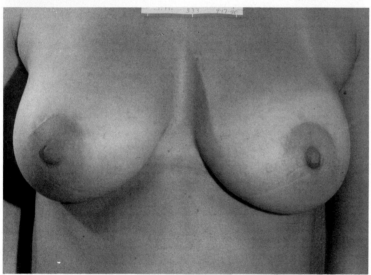

B

Figure 1.10. A third example of treatment of breast ptosis by crescent mastopexy combined with breast prostheses. **(A)** Before treatment; **(B)** after treatment.

ment, even with saline prostheses (as noted in Chapter 10). The major disappointment with the saline prosthesis is not the low deflation rate, but the often visible rippling. Overinflation has not eliminated much of this problem, but the rippling is frequently visible in the lower quadrants.

In Chapter 10, on breast repair, reference is made to the use of autologous tissue and capsule to "patch" these thinned areas where ripples are more visible. Submuscular placement will conceal superior wrinkles, but in my experience and those of surgeons with whom I correspond, visible rippling in the upper part of the breast is a rare

phenomenon unless there has been some saline loss.

The internal repair of the stretched-out breast with either resection of tissue or, more com-

> *Why the Circle When Implants Are Removed?*
> Repair ptosis
> Minimal new scar (patient is already upset!)
> Technical: Smaller size breast (B cup)
>   Reflect skin, infold

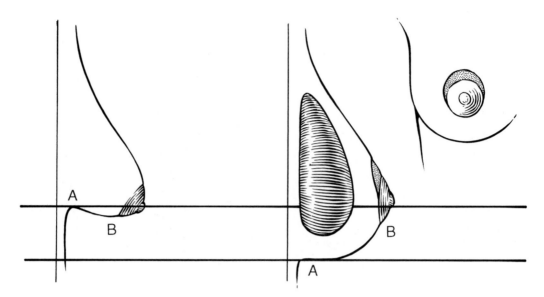

Figure 1.11. Schematic depiction of excessive lowering of the inframammary fold.

monly, left-to-right cross-over reinforcement, further conceals the prosthesis.

In a smaller number of patients who require internal repair the areola has descended and a complete circle deepithelialization is performed as described in Chapter 7 on mastopexy.

In certain patients (e.g., patient K.V. in Figure 1.12A–D) circumareolar mastopexy is not required because the breast prosthesis gives elevation to the nipple-areolar complex. This is a "pseudo-Snoopy" deformity. Breast tissue is primarily beneath the areola but there is also a moderate amount of distribution in other quadrants. Using the short periareolar incision allows us to physically expand this soft tissue. The weight of the implant continues the expansion. Patient K.V. has maintained her configuration by consistently wearing a brassiere and has not required further uplift or reinforcement in 12 years.

It is obviously easier to control scar visibility with a short incision such as this, rather than with a circular incision.

Many patients request that their nipples be made smaller, but I generally discourage this. Circumareolar techniques are useful for making the nipple smaller, but the scar is not as natural in appearance as the blending noted here.

Breast prostheses used in 1979 were quite stiff and heavy compared to the ones that are in use today. The short periareolar incision was roughly twice the length of those required for modern saline implants. The incision is woven in a wiggly manner along the junction line between taut, unpigmented skin and the pigmented skin of the areola. The wiggly incision prevents scar contracture, which would increase the visibility of the incision. It also visually breaks the junction between pigmented and nonpigmented skin. When the scar is still in the red phase, it blends with the areola. When the scar finally blurs into white it blends easily with the adjacent skin. In black patients it is best to deepithelialize the edge of the skin and allow the scar to overlap, thus creating a more natural junction line in that 2-mm space just below the actual incision.

Patient C.M., depicted in Figure 1.13, required elevation of only one areola. Upper areolar incisions do not blend as easily as the subareolar incision. The skin and soft tissue excision does, however, allow a greater degree of balancing. The excision of this wedge of tissue (the crescent mastopexy) is combined with lowering of the inframammary fold so that one obtains both the internal up-push of the nipple-areolar complex from the implant, and the actual physical repositioning. This was a forerunner of the Toledo triangle maneuver, which is described in Chapter 7 on circumareolar mastopexy and reduction.

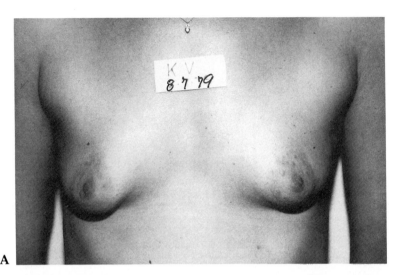

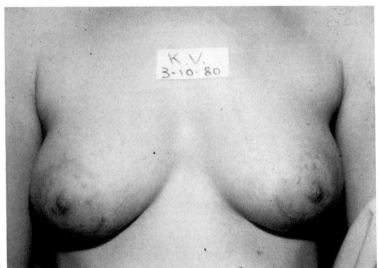

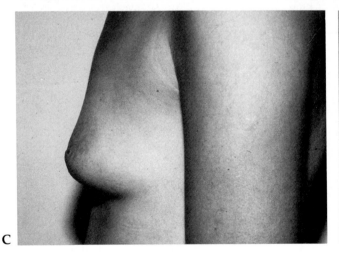

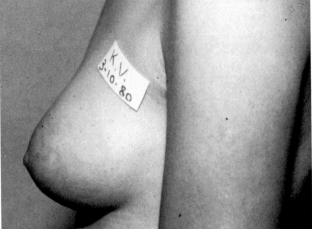

Figure 1.12. Insertion of breast prostheses elevates the nipple-areolar complex sufficiently, without the need for mastopexy. **(A, C)** Before prosthetic insertion; **(B, D)** after insertion.

Figure 1.13. When only one breast is treated (in this patient the right areola was elevated), scarring becomes more noticeable relative to the untreated breast. Here, a subareolar incision yielded optimal results.

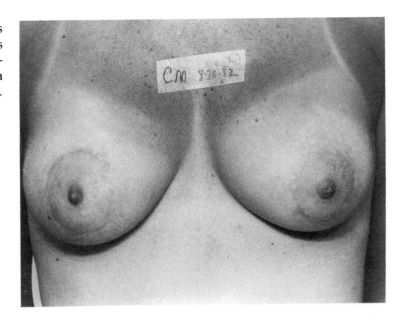

Category C-4—A Greater Degree of Ptosis

Obviously, there are fewer problems if ptosis can be disguised by the preceding maneuvers, which are referred to as "illusion" mastopexies, or in category C-3 patients by repairing an overstretched breast and repositioning or removing a breast prosthesis (Figure 1.14).

Solving the problems of "internal" mastopexy and reduction involves a number of technical maneuvers to prevent the areolar expansion and breast flattening illustrated in the earlier literature (see references in Chapter 2). The problems are those of creating the internal mound, and assuring that the reduced nipple and areola will stay at a predetermined position and expand only an acceptable size.

In the small mastopexy, the inframammary position must be securely sutured at an acceptable level. One problem was solved by anchoring this tissue after the completion of the Erol-type infolding. The infolding must be with multiple lattice-like sutures to ensure that stretching does not occur with subsequent flattening of the cone.

Adding liposuction, even in the smaller reductions and mastopexies, was popularized by Luiz Toledo. This solved the problem of the rounded ball shape with fullness at the superior edge of the areola.

An aggressive use of liposuction in the larger breast solved the problem or irregular distribution of breast parenchyma, because the major resection is in the inferior quadrant.

Creating the cone in large and small reductions is no longer a problem if one considers the operation as a subcutaneous Pitanguy wedge resection (Figure 1.15). Simply closing the wedge is only the beginning, however. As illustrated in more detail in Chapter 9, the wedge is removed, the breast is coned, and the excessive tissue at the base of the cone is trimmed away until the desired shape is obtained.

With the circular removal of skin, the areola tends to remain in the center of the circle rather than at the superior edge, which would give it a normal positioning at the tip of the cone. Removing a wedge of subcutaneous tissue and breast prior to cone creation allows us to set the nipple at its predetermined position. This wedge resection (the Toledo triangle or the Texas diamond) is an anchoring maneuver that is completed before skin advancement.

Create a Cone Shape Subcutaneously
1. Infold, or
2. Resect, or
3. Overlap, and add a new implant

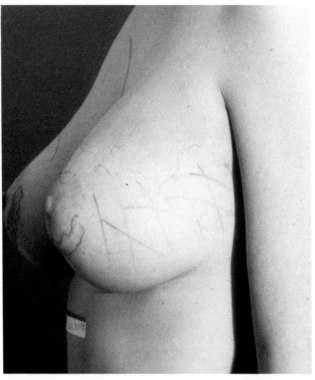

A

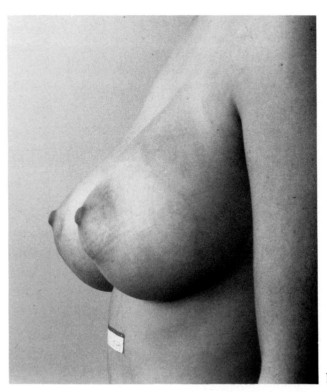

B

Figure 1.14. This patient was distressed not only by the extremely wide periareolar scars, the thick fibrocystic encapsular changes laterally, but also by the rapid descent of her breasts **(A)**. Her surgery had been performed in another city by a surgeon who is not in our specialty. The visible hatch marks from the incision closure were eliminated by the meticulous subcuticular closure described in Chapter 10 on breast repair. The overstretch of the lower half of the breasts was repaired at the time of prosthetic replacement. The left-to-right overfolding was performed subcutaneously, allowing us to restore the natural contour and force the areolae to a more upward position. This patient maintained the correction for 4 years **(B)** until pregnancy created additional stretching, which has subsequently been repaired.

Louis Benelli contributed a major technical innovation in his presentations on the "round block" technique, now used in reductions as well. Deepithelialization of the circle yields firmer tissue to which to anchor bites of the circumareolar suture. Since the initial description, there is an addition of crossing sutures to the Benelli circular suture technique. We now use both Benelli's nonabsorbable suture and a more superficial circular absorbable suture, to eliminate the problem of spitting or distortion from knot failure.

The circumareolar mastopexy or reduction is definitely a hands-on operation that appeals to the creativity of plastic surgeons. With the tech-

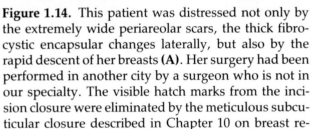

Mastopexy
Erol—Infold, little or no skin excision
Benelli—Large deepithelialization, circle suture
Brazilians—Liposuction, dermis/silicone slings
Texas—Larger size (adding prosthesis)
    Lesser deepithelialized ring
    Diamond lift
    Overlap for reinforcement

nical maneuvers described in greater detail in subsequent chapters, many potentially unsatisfactory results can be avoided and these same maneuvers may be applied in other situations as well.

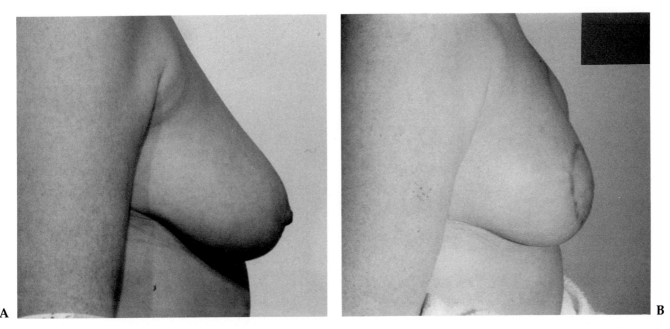

A B

Figure 1.15. An example of a subcutaneous Pitanguy wedge resection.

Advantages of the Circumareolar Approach

Adrien Aiache

There is definitely a need for circumareolar procedures. By definition, the circumareolar approach allows a repositioning of the nipple-areolar complex with a subcutaneous reshaping of the glandular portion of the breast. In contrast to the "skin brassiere" techniques, the skin does not play a role in maintaining the shape of the breast. Instead, the internal cone development, tissue reduction, and fixation at the new inframammary fold play the major roles. In contrast to the skeletonized pedicles described in the plastic surgery literature, the entire breast serves as a pedicle for the nipple-areolar complex, and the newly created mound is repositioned. In theory, this would preserve sensation to a greater degree, in addition to preserving the ductal structures. In the younger patient, breast feeding may not be possible even with the thicker bipedicle generated by the McKissock technique. Breast feeding is not compromised by the circumareolar technique.

The major advantages of the circumareolar technique are the avoidance of scars on the unpredictable breast skin (Figure 1.6). For the younger patient in our practice, scars are a major concern. Concern about scars has been blithely

> *The Circumareolar Technique*
> Mastopexy—Areolar lift?
>   Add prosthesis?
> Reduction—Moderate, or larger (younger age group)
> Repair—Overstretch group
>   Prosthesis removal group

dismissed by many of our colleagues, but this attitude is not shared by most patients when they are offered procedural choices. In all but extreme ptosis with parenchymal loss, skin damage, or the massively hypertrophied breast, the circumareolar technique should be presented as a reasonable alternative.

The circumareolar technique for gynecomastia is no longer a choice. New developments in sharp and blunt suction have replaced even the traditional small circle excisional procedures. "Controlled scraping," as well as sharp-tipped and blunt-tipped liposuction cannulas, are employed. As noted in the excellent review by Gary Rosenburg,[5] these procedures are now applicable for all cases of gynecomastia.

From a practical, aesthetic viewpoint, the circumareolar mammoplasty presents a distinct advantage. The limited extent of the scar and its specific location around the areola allows a young woman to wear a small bathing suit top or any brassiere without the fear of exhibiting the large scars secondary to the inverted T closure used in most mammoplasty techniques.

From a security standpoint, the circumareolar mammoplasty technique is not associated with any of the skin sloughing associated with the inverted anchor closure technique. Although circumareolar slough can be seen in the circular scar if the suturing is sufficiently extensive and tight, it is rare and limited to the scar only. The circular technique of undermining the skin has proved safe if the skin is left relatively thick with underlying fat.

If they are necessary, revisions are also limited to the same scar, which is easily hidden even by the smallest brassiere as opposed to the revision techniques in the inverted scar that could infringe medially and laterally, preventing complete coverage of the scars by the bra.

References

1. Bartels RJ, Strickland DM, Douglas WM: A new mastopexy operation for mild or moderate breast ptosis. Plast Reconstr Surg 57:687, 1976.
2. Davidson BA: Concentric circle operation for massive gynecomastia to excise the redundant skin. Plast Reconstr Surg 63:350, 1979.
3. Erol O, Spira M: A mastopexy technique for mild to moderate ptosis. Plast Reconstr Surg 65:603, 1980.
4. Lejour M: Reduction mammoplasty by suction alone: Discussion. Plast Reconstr Surg 92:1286, 1993.
5. Rosenburg G: Surgical correction for gynecomastia: An update. In: *Advances in Plastic and Reconstructive Surgery*, Vol. 10. C. V. Mosby-Year Book Medical Publishers, Chicago, 1994, pp. 285–334.
6. Wilkinson TS: Gel mammary augmentation via minimal periareolar incision. In: *Symposium on Aesthetic Surgery of the Breast*, Vol. 44. Owsley TQ, Peterson RA (Eds.). C. V. Mosby, St. Louis, Missouri, 1978, pp. 312–317.
7. Wilkinson TS: In: *Aesthetic Breast Surgery*, Vol. 7. Georgiade NG (Ed.). Williams & Wilkins, Baltimore, 1983, pp. 71–86.
8. Wilkinson TS: In: *The Art of Aesthetic Surgery*, Vol. 127. Louis JR (Ed.). Little, Brown, Boston, 1989, pp. 833–836.
9. Puckett CL, Meyer DH, Reinisch JF: Crescent mastopexy and augmentation. Plast Reconstr Surg 75:533–538, 1985.

History and Overview

Adrien Aiache

As is often the case, a technique for circumareolar excision was imagined by a young plastic surgery resident, Dr. Enrique Rossell from Guatemala, who was in training with Dr. Richard Stark of New York. A relative lack of experience and knowledge can sometimes produce ideas that sound impossible, even insane, to more seasoned colleagues, who find later that it opens new vistas in the field. Such an occurrence took place while I was a medical student: a young student asked our professor if bowed legs could not be straightened by cutting the bones in many areas and fixing them on skewer-type wiring not unlike a shish kebab. This immediately raised the laughter of the whole class and it made him look ridiculous. Yet Ilizarov was probably of a similar age in 1948 and already thinking of a similar technique that is now a breakthrough in orthopedic surgery.

History of the Circumareolar Procedure

Adrien Aiache

The history of the circumareolar procedure begins in the early part of this century. In 1924 Höllander[1] first excised skin in the supraareolar area, creating what is now called the "crescent" areolar lift. He was followed by Joseph in 1925,[2] Cesari in 1927,[3] and Noel et al. in 1928[4] with different types of supraareolar excisions of skin in order to lift the nipple in a ptotic breast. Other reports were by Glasmer in 1930[5] and Eitner in 1932.[6] These authors were elevating only the areola. Breast reduction or elevation was performed with other types of incisions, such as the axillary lift of Höllander. It was only in 1969 that the first modern attempt at a "doughnut mastopexy" was presented.[7] Ulrich Hinderer began his technique on a moderate number of cases, warning that the technique should be limited to minimal hypertrophies and minimal ptotic cases. His complications of wide scars, breast flattening,[8,9] and areolar expansion have been almost but not completely eliminated today. A more acceptable circumareolar mastopexy was the Rossell and Stark presentation at the American Society of Plastic and Reconstructive Surgeons annual meeting in 1973.[10] These authors were apparently unaware of Hinderer's[8] or An-

drews'[11] publications. This was followed by Bartels et al.,[12] who used a circle procedure in small mastopexies and reported the problems in the larger breasts. Soon other reports, including those by Vecchione,[13] Rees and Aston,[14] Bass,[15] Davidson,[16] and Erol and Spira[17] (Erol being the father of modern circumareolar surgery), emphasized reconstructing the mammary mounds, although this had been mentioned by Hinderer in his original article. The concept of reconstructing the breast mound did not find wide acceptance initially. The procedure was largely rejected because of the almost universal complications of poor breast shape and scar stretching. Techniques producing a flat "pancake" shape but better control of areolar size were presented by Gruber and Jones,[18] Teimourian and Adams,[19] Saad,[20] Peled et al.,[21] and Felício.[22,23]

Wilkinson[24] and Puckett et al.[25] emphasized the procedures that created the illusion of mastopexy by combining a crescent excision for areolar lift with lowering of the inframammary fold to accommodate a breast prosthesis. Wilkinson reported scar hypertrophy problems with the circumareolar procedure in 1978, and again in a lecture series in 1985. Louis Benelli also presented a series, as did Luiz Toledo in 1985, showing better scar control, but in smaller breasts without prosthetic augmentation. A review of these cases shows lesser degrees of scarring but, unfortunately, a flatter than desired breast shape. The concept of "round block" shaping,[26,27] the circular tension-relieving nonabsorbable "Benelli suture," and sutures anchored to deepithelialized dermis stimulated the evolution of mastopexy. The interest in this technique is now very keen; the many authors expanding on the concept, and who continue the quest for perfection and reliability[28–33] by quantifying the amount of skin to be undermined and the amount of breast tissue to be either resected or plicated, plus other technical changes, reflect the willingness of surgeons to attack the problems inherent in any reshaping of the human female breast. Whether one undermines the entire gland or the entire breast skin (but not both together!), uses criss-crossed or circular advancing and tension-relieving sutures, or adds liposuction as a major or minor component of the procedure reflects the technique of the individual surgeon in a valuable procedure that is still evolving. The complications of breast descent, scar widening, or areolar distortion that accompany a certain percentage of cases of breast mastopexy and reduction will probably never be completely eliminated, owing to the inherent structure and individual variations of the female breast. They occur in superior pedicle, inferior pedicle, and double pedicle surgeries, as well as in the circumareolar procedures. As our experience progresses, and further technical advances are added, we should see the current trend of fewer and fewer revisions continue.

References

1. Holländer E: Die Operation der Mammahypertrophie und der haenge Brust. Dtsch Med Wochenschr 41:1400, 1924.
2. Joseph J: Zur Operation der Hypertrophisehen haenge Brust. Dtsch Med Wochenschr 51:1103, 1925.
3. Cesari: 1927. Upwards transposition of the nipple-areolar complex.
4. Noel A, Lopez, Martinez M: Noveaux procedes chirugicaux de correction du prolapsus mammaire. Arch Franco Belge Chir 31:138, 1928.
5. Glasmer E: Die Formfehler und die plastichen Operationen der veiblicen Brust. Ferdinand Enk Verlag, Stuttgart, 1930.
6. Eitner E 1932. Superior crescent nipple-areolar complex excision with superior breast tissue excision. Julius Springer, Wien, 1932.
7. Hinderer U: Primera Experiencia con una Nueva Tecnica de Mastoplastia para Ptosis Ligeres. Presented at the Sixth National Reunion of Spanish Society of Plastic and Reparative Surgery, Madrid, October 29–31, 1969.
8. Hinderer U: Mammary plastic modeling with superficial dermopexy and retromammary dermopexy. Revista Esp Cir Plast 5(1):65, 1972.
9. Hinderer U: Reduction and augmentation mammaplasty, remodeling mammaplasty with superficial and retromammary mastopexy. Internat. Micr J Aesth Plast Surg E, 1972.
10. Rossell E, Stark RB: Circumareolar Mastopexy. Presented at the American Society of Plastic and Reconstructive Surgeons Convention, October 23, 1976, Hollywood, Florida.
11. Andrews JM, Yshisuki MM, Martins DMSF, Ramos RR: An areolar approach for reduction mammoplasty. Br J Plast Surg 28:166, 1975.
12. Bartels RJ, Strickland DM, Douglas WM: A new mastopexy operation for mild or moderate breast ptosis. Plast Reconstr Surg 57:687, 1976.
13. Vecchione TR: A method for re-contouring the domed nipple. Plast Reconstr Surg 57:30, 1976.
14. Rees TD and Aston SJ: The tuberous breast. Clin Plast Surg 3:339, 1976.
15. Bass CP: Herniated areolar complex. Ann Plast Surg 1:402, 1978.
16. Davidson BA: Concentric circle operation for massive gynecomastia to excise the redundant skin. Plast Reconstr Surg 63:350, 1979.
17. Erol O, Spira M: A mastopexy technique for mild to moderate ptosis. Plast Reconstr Surg 65:609, 1980.
18. Gruber RB, Jones HW: The "Donut" mastopexy: Indications and complications. Plast Reconstr Surg 65:34, 1980.
19. Teimourian B, Adams MN: Surgical correction of the tuberous breast. Ann Plast Surg 10:190, 1983.
20. Saad MN: An extended circumareolar incision for breast augmentation and gynecomastia. Aesth Plast Surg 7:127, 1983.
21. Peled I, Zagher V, Wexler MR: Purse string for reduction and closure of skin defects. Ann Plast Surg 14:465, 1985.
22. Felício Y: Mammoplastia de reduction con solo una incision periareolar. Revista Ibezo Latino Americane de Cizurgia Plastica 12:245, 1986.
23. Felício Y: Periareolar reduction mammoplasty. Plast Reconstr Surg 88:789, 1991.
24. Wilkinson TS: Gel mammary augmentation via minimal periareolar incision (synopsis). In: Aesthetic Surgery of the Breast, Vol. 18. Owsley JQ, Peterson RA (Eds). C. V. Mosby, St. Louis, 1978, p. 312.
25. Puckett CL, Meyer DH, Reinish JF: Crescent mastopexy and augmentation. Plast Reconstr Surg 75:533, 1985.
26. Benelli L: Technique de plastic mammaire "round block." Rev Chir Esth Langue Francaise. 13(50):7, 1988.

27. Benelli L: A new periareolar mammoplasty: The "round block" technique. Aesth Plast Surg 14:93, 1990.
28. Bustos RA: Mammoplastia reduction con cicatriz periareolar. Transactas VII Congrese Ibero Latino Americano de Cirurgia Plastica. Cartagena de Indias, 1988.
29. Gasperoni C, Salgarelto M, Gargani J: Experience and technical refinements in the "doughnut" mastopexy with augmentation mammoplasty. Aesth Plast Surg 12:111, 1988.
30. Toledo LS, Matsudo PK: Mammoplasty using liposuction and the periareolar incision. Aesth Plast Surg 13:9, 1989.
31. Goes JCS: Periareolar mammoplasty, double skin technique. 4:111, 1991; Rev Bras Cir Plast 4(23):55, 1989.
32. Spear SL, Kassan M, Little JW: Guidelines in concentric mastopexy. Plast Reconstr Surg 85:961, 1990.
33. Passot R. Plastie mammaire periareolaire avec pedicule inferieur et ancrage cutaneo dermique areolaire correcteurs. Rev Chir Aesth XVI 63:31, 1991.

Other Periareolar Techniques That Have Influenced Us

Luiz S. Toledo

The shape of the breast is determined by the balance between its contents, gland and fat, and the skin that covers it. The periareolar approach, widely used by Davidson[1] and others for excision of glandular pathologies, or for insertion of mammary implants, has lately been reintroduced as a technique for reduction mammoplasties and mastopexies.

Early attempts to achieve mammary reduction and mastopexy by the periareolar approach faced three problems: (1) late widening of the areola by the centrifugal action of the skin, (2) flattening of the breast shape, and (3) premature postoperative ptosis due to a lack of support tissue. The ideal shape and scar will not be obtained unless the weight of the breast is proportional to the quality of the skin. If the breast remains large and heavy with loose skin, ptosis will result. If the skin is too tight, we will see areolar enlargement or hypertrophic scarring.

We have compiled several periareolar mammoplasty techniques and studied their differences in an attempt to understand the discrepancy in the individual results obtained. Our questions concerned the originality of the technique, the difference in technique between one surgeon and another, where their influences originated, advantages and disadvantages, and indications and contraindications as seen through their eyes.

Hinderer (Madrid) believes his technique, published in 1969,[2,3] is original. He says it differs from the techniques published by Joseph (1925),[4] Cesary (1927),[4a] and Noel (1928),[5] all of which remove skin above the areola in one or several stages, and by Eitner (1932), who removes an oval ring of full-thickness periareolar skin, with skin dissection and resection of the superior transverse keel of the gland. Our bibliographical research confirmed that the first report of a "doughnut" technique was presented[2] and published by Hinderer in 1969[3] and 1972,[6] a "periareolar dermopexy technique with retromammary mastopexy," in order to elevate the gland and the nipple-areolar complex (Figure 2.1).

Most authors point out that the main advantage of this approach is the existence of only one periareolar scar. The disadvantages of the Hinderer technique are the widening of the scar, and the flattening of the nipple-areolar complex (Figure 2.2). Hinderer indicates the technique for moderate ptotic breasts, moderate ptotic hypoplastic breasts, and tuberous breasts (all

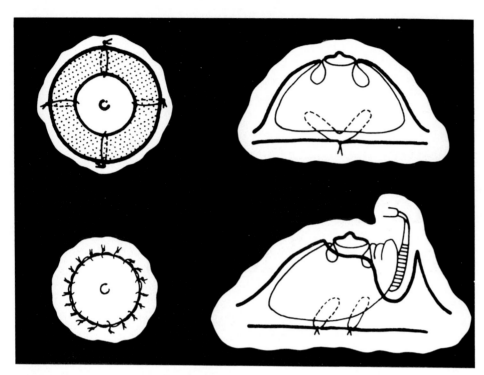

Figure 2.1. Original drawing of Hinderer "doughnut" technique,[3] or "periareolar dermopexy with retromammary mastopexy." *Top:* The infraareolar skin is dissected from the gland toward the retromammary space. *Bottom:* Nonabsorbable sutures are used to elevate the gland and achieve projection of the breast cone.

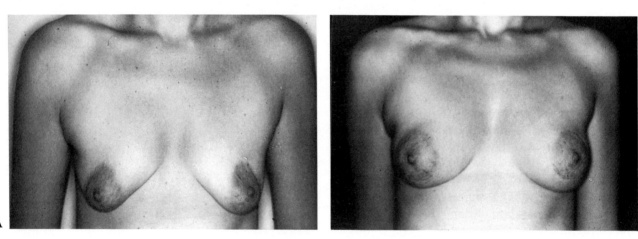

A   B

Figure 2.2. (A) Preoperative and **(B)** postoperative result with Hinderer's doughnut technique in a ptotic breast. There is widening and flattening of the areola and widening of the periareolar scar.

treated by the addition of subpectoral breast implants), as well as moderate ptotic breasts with minor hypertrophy (treated by the addition of a Pitanguy keel breast resection).[7] He contraindicates it for moderate and large hypertrophies. When the ptosis and hypertrophy are moderate (approximately 250 cm^3), he adds a vertical scar and infraareolar V excision. Hinderer is pleased with the periareolar mastopexy only when an additional retromammary mastopexy procedure is used in conjunction. He performs a maximum 250-g resection per breast, believing that short scar techniques should not be used at the cost of the aesthetic result and postoperative stability. Breast projection with his technique is good in cases of minor hypertrophies (up to 100 cm^3), hypoplasias, and tuberous breasts (with implants).

Andrews, Yshizuki, Martins, and Ramos (São Paulo, Brazil) described in 1975[8] an areolar approach for breast reduction, which they had used in ten selected women under 40 years old, who had good skin elasticity and were physically active. The circular incision is actually intraareolar, which becomes periareolar after adjacent skin removal. The mastopexy is performed according to Arié's technique (1957)[9] (without the vertical skin resection), infolding the gland and securing it to the pectoral muscle and to the rib periosteum. The indications are to correct ptosis and small to medium hypertrophy. At the time of publication (1975) more than 90% of their patients were young active women under 40 years of age, the ideal candidates for this technique.

Bartels, Strickland, and Douglas (Orlando, FL) described in 1976[10] a mastopexy technique, with or without augmentation, for mild to moderate ptosis that is based on the circumferential excision of skin around the areola. The areolar size can be reduced during augmentation, leaving a single circular scar at the junction of skin and areola. Two circular incision lines are made, the inner incision being located on the border of the areola. The second circular (or oval) incision is positioned to keep the nipple at the crest of the breast cone. The distance from the areola to the inframammary fold should not exceed 5 cm (or possibly 4 cm in a smaller woman). This distance locates the inferior limit of the outer skin incision.

We think this procedure is still useful for young patients with mild to moderate ptosis. This type of mastopexy is based purely on skin excision; the gland is not treated. The main problem associated with this technique is areolar enlargement.

Erol (Istanbul, Turkey) and Spira (Houston) published in 1980[11] a circumareolar mastopexy, the main target of which was to obtain a conical breast shape by molding the breast gland using a "rotation-invagination" maneuver. Through a 360° circumareolar incision the skin of the entire breast is undermined under the superficial fascia. The areola remains attached to the mammary gland with its vascularity deriving from the perforating vessels of the gland. By means of a rotation-invagination procedure that can be repeated two or three times, the breast is sutured into a conical shape, correcting the ptosis. There is no skin excision.

The treatment for the different types of ptosis and hypertrophies has been divided into 11 groups by Erol (1992),[12] according to the type of problem. By following his classification, results are more predictable and suitable. Erol notes that the duration of a good result will depend on each patient and breast type.

Felício (Fortaleza, Brazil) reports no influences in the initial development of her technique (1984)[13] or later.[14,15] Glandular resection is circular, beveled in the shape of a cake slice, and removed from around the gland, leaving the gland and the nipple-areolar complex pedicled to the pectoral muscle. The disadvantage of this technique is again the enlargement of the areolar scar. Her indications are ptosis and to reduce up to 50% of breast hypertrophy. For ptosis a prosthesis is added.

Bustos, Loureiro, and Thame (São Paulo, Brazil) reported in 1985[16] a mammoplasty procedure influenced by McKissock[17] and Jurado,[18] and involving a periareolar incision and a trilobulated flap with an inferior pedicle and a periareolar approach. This technique, which is based on the pathophysiological mechanisms of the breast alterations and on the neurovascular anatomy of the anterior thoracic wall, is indicated for young patients with ptosis and moderate to severe hypertrophy, up to 500 g per breast, or the associa-

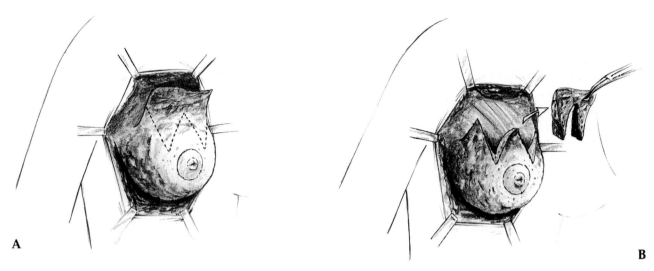

Figure 2.3. The Bustos technique: A trilobulated flap **(A)** with an inferior pedicle and a periareolar approach and **(B)** resection of gland in the upper quadrants.

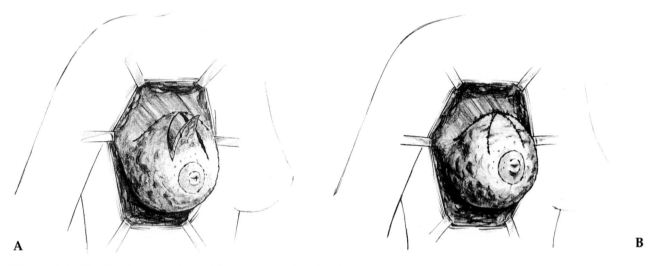

Figure 2.4. The Bustos technique: Mastopexy and reduction.

tion of both. The contraindications are for older patients, patients with ptosis and mammary hypoplasia, and for patients with extreme hypertrophy or hypertrophy associated with ptosis.[19] Postoperative ptosis is avoided with the inclusion of a silicone supporting sheet (or more recently polyurethane)[20] placed around the breast in the subcutaneous layer, anchoring it to the anterior pectoral fascia (Figure 2.3).

This allows for good protection and durability of the result. The other difference is the resection of gland in the upper quadrants. The main disad-

vantage of the technique is the use of a foreign body and its inherent complications. Bustos believes the sheet, inserted as a supporting device, keeps the shape, prevents recurrence of ptosis, and leads to volumetric fitness of the integument, which now covers and no longer supports the gland (Figure 2.4).

No pathological processes were observed as a result of use of the prosthesis. The silicone sheet did not interfere with manual or mammographic examinations during the follow-up period. Bustos continues to be pleased with the reduction of

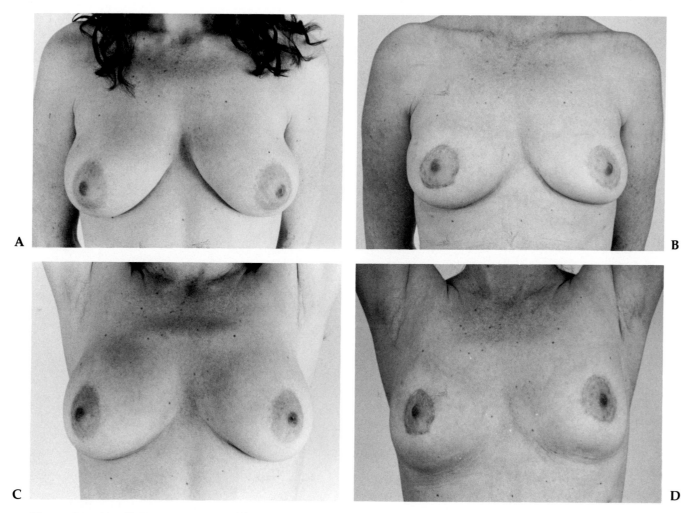

Figure 2.5. (A, C) Preoperative and (B, D) postoperative result of breast reduction and mastopexy using the Bustos technique, with the polyurethane sheet.

breast volume and the mastopexy obtained. The reduction and mastopexy are easily performed using the Bustos technique and a beautiful breast shape can be obtained (Figure 2.5).

In the techniques that utilize the inverted T incision with skin removal, the resultant scar acts as a "skin brassiere," or "dermal belt," holding the breast in place and helping avoid early ptosis, a problem with the periareolar technique. The dermal belt is substituted in the Bustos technique by the polyurethane sheet, objectionable in some cases, when the patient cannot be followed closely during the first six postoperative months. The controversy, as with all alloplastic inclusions, is the possibility of infection, rejection, or extrusion as in the objection to the polyurethane-covered breast prosthesis. I personally have not yet seen complications with the polyurethane sheet, as utilized for the last 2 years. I have, however, removed six pairs of silicone sheets from patients who underwent the Bustos technique, although not performed by Bustos himself. The complications included skin irregularities and noticeable retraction, especially with arm movements (Figure 2.6). The allegation that the inclusion of this fine sheet would interfere with the examination of the breast by mammography has not been proved.

Toledo and Matsudo (São Paulo, Brazil) presented their findings at the International Society

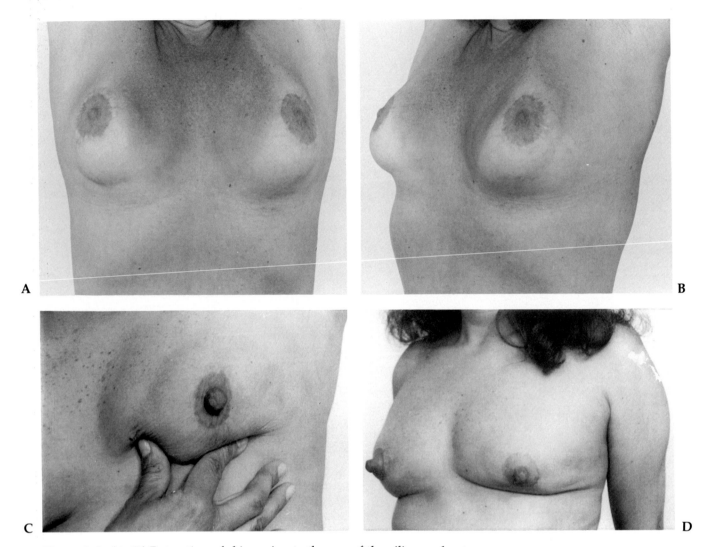

Figure 2.6. (A–D) Retraction of skin owing to the use of the silicone sheet.

for Aesthetic Plastic Surgery (ISAPS) meeting in New York (1987)[21] (subsequently published in 1989[22]). With this technique, selected breasts can be reduced by liposuction, the mastopexy being performed through a periareolar incision. Problems appeared when we attempted to treat breasts that were too big, too flaccid, or both. In these cases the results lacked projection in the shape of the breast and showed a widening of the areola (see Chapter 7).

Toledo published in 1989 a combination of syringe liposuction and periareolar incision,[23] showing the removal of a pyramid or a prism of gland from the upper pole of the breast to elevate

the areola; this was followed in 1990 by a publication describing 4 years of experience with this technique[24] (see Chapter 7).

An attempted solution for the late enlarging of the areola was published by Peled, Zagher, and Wexler (Jerusalem, Israel) in 1985[25]; they conceived of a purse-string suture for reduction and closure of skin defects, among them the suture of a periareolar incision for treatment of gynecomastia. Peled believes the purse-string suture is original "in some ways" and he uses it in selected cases for reduction of areolar size and minor reduction mammoplasty. The purse string avoids the stretching of the areola, but this permanent

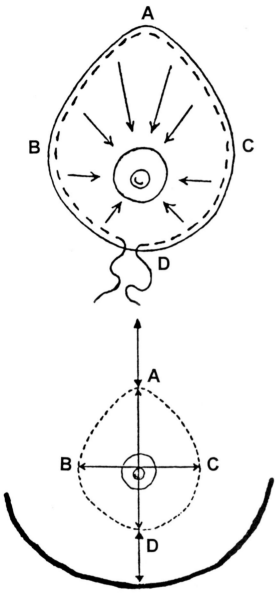

Figure 2.7. The Benelli purse-string stitch. *Bottom:* Preoperative markings. *Top:* Placement of single purse-string suture.

stitch is also the main disadvantage of the technique. Peled usually reduces very large breasts, a limitation for reduction and mastopexy using his periareolar approach. He is not pleased with the reduction of breast volume and the mastopexy obtained through the periareolar technique. He prefers the inferior pedicle technique.

Benelli (Paris) proposed in 1988[26] and 1990[27] a similar permanent periareolar circling suture

(Figure 2.8). In all types of mammoplasty, one main objective is to limit the scar. The scar in the submammary fold is visible, particularly when one is lying down. The ideal result would be to confine the scar to the periareolar area. He suggests a crossed mastopexy in the lower hemisphere of the breast to improve its shape. He states that his technique, the "round block," should act as a keystone supporting the mammary cone. The keystone lies in the dermo-dermic, glandulo-glandular, and glandulo-musculo-periosteal unions fixed definitively with unabsorbable suture, by a criss-cross mastopexy, and by a circular unabsorbable suture of woven Nylon (Figure 2.7) included in the periareolar circular dermo-dermic scar block. He uses his technique in numerous types of breast surgery, including cases of ptosis or hypertrophy, and in cases of hypotrophy, when the use of the round block technique permits easy access for insertion of the prosthesis as it simultaneously corrects ptosis. In cases of tumoral excision, the round block should produce a discreet scar and a more regular breast contour.

In 1989 we started using a Mersilene 0 periareolar purse-string stitch in our patients,[24] after seeing Benelli's results. Our impression is that the stitch does maintain the size of the areola, but is not free of its own problems. Depending on the amount of skin resected, the stitch might constrict the breast, flattening it and provoking a round shape with an unnatural projection of the areola. Some patients have presented an allergy to the thread and had it removed. One patient submitted to a periareolar mastopexy with augmentation, and showed a very good 6-month postoperative result. At 12 months the thread on the left areola had broken, provoking an enlargement of the areola even at this late stage (Figure 2.9).

Wilkinson (San Antonio, TX) in 1991,[28] as opposed to Benelli, advocates a double periareolar suture, one of Mersilene 2-0 at a distance from the areola, and another of 2-0 Dexon in the subcuticular position at the areolar edge. Wilkinson states this double-suture technique has largely eliminated the spreading of the areola in the postoperative period, for him the major problem of

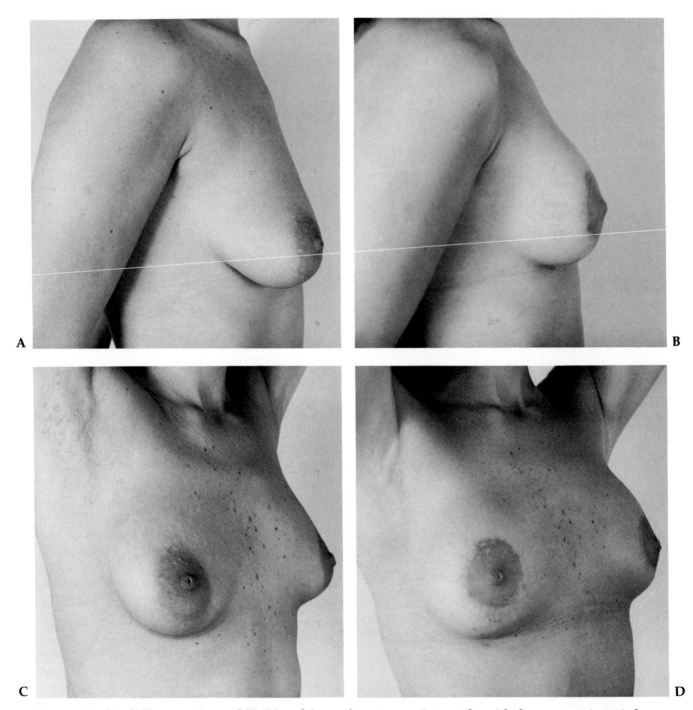

Figure 2.8. **(A, C)** Preoperative and **(B, D)** and 6-month postoperative results with the purse-string stitch.

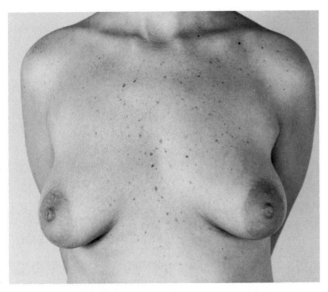
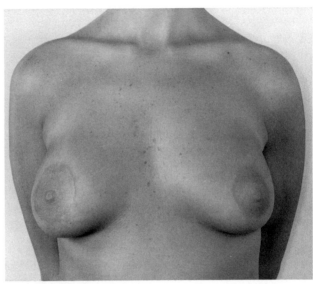

A

B

Figure 2.9. Same patient as in Figure 2.8, but at 12 months postoperatively, showing late areolar enlargement after the breaking of the purse-string stitch.

doughnut mastopexy. For patients with large implants where the lower breast has stretched out, the double reinforcement internally has certainly repaired the damage without skin excision scars. For Wilkinson,[29] circumareolar breast reduction became the procedure of choice for his younger patients. He now performs his technique on patients with a greater degree of ptosis, patients with less satisfactory skin elasticity, and patients with larger breasts, avoiding the troublesome inframammary fold scars, with less of a risk to areolar circulation.

Hinderer[30] added the Benelli round block suture, and a second block suture, to produce an anterior herniation of the nipple-areolar complex to prevent the widening of the areola and flattening of the nipple-areolar complex (Figure 2.10).

Ersek and Ersek (Austin, TX) published in 1991[31] their 10-year experience with what they call a circular cinching stitch, used for minimum mastopexies, augmentation, or special circumstances. One special circumstance in which the technique was applied was the 420-cm³ augmentation and areolar reduction of an exotic dancer, a profession that requires minimal scarring on the breasts. Wilkinson and Ersek's stitch differs from Peled's and Benelli's because they suture the

larger outer circle to the areola, whereas Benelli places a continuous stitch only in the external circle, which he reduces as a purse string to the desired areolar diameter and then sutures to the areola with separate stitches.

Goes (São Paulo, Brazil) described in 1989[32] a technique utilizing transposition of flaps with a periareolar approach. He uses it for the treatment of ptosis and medium hypertrophies of the breast. He employed the deepithelialized skin around the areola to fashion the breast and stabilize its shape. He based his technique on the reports of Ribeiro (Niterói, Brazil), in 1989,[33] of mammaplasties with inferior pedicle flaps and inverted T incisions. Goes believes in the principle that breast shape is ensured by its contents and that skin will retract and adjust to it.

Spear, Kassan, and Little (Washington, DC) in 1990[34] published guidelines for concentric mastopexy for patients with mild skin excess and a large areola. They treat mild nipple ptosis, glandular ptosis, and areolar asymmetry, as well as the tuberous breast. Their technique is contraindicated in cases of severe skin excess.

Spear[35] believes the technique to be original in some ways; the main advantage is safety, and the main disadvantages are the standard risks of

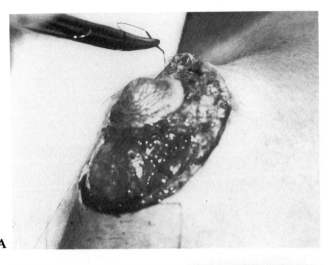

A

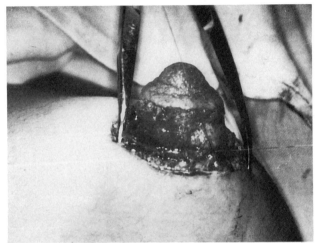

B

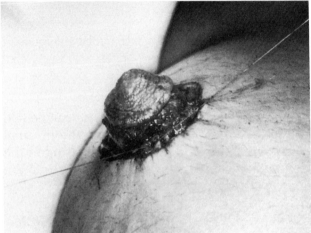

C

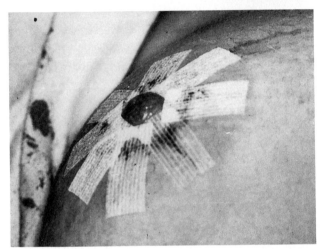

D

Figure 2.10. Hinderer's double round block technique. **(A, B)** The first suture of Tri-cron 3-0 is placed at 2 cm around the areola and adjusted to a diameter of approximately 3.5 cm, to produce anterior herniation of the nipple-areolar complex. **(C, D)** The Benelli "round block" suture, with Tri-cron 3-0, to prevent widening of the scar. Skin is closed intradermally with Surgilene 4-0 and Micropore dressing is applied for skin adaptation.

flattening. Generally he is pleased with the shape and breast projection obtained by their technique. The limitations for reduction and mastopexy using their technique are when nipple height does not have to be raised significantly (1 or 2 cm). Their paper recommends some arithmetic and geometric calculations. Early disappointment has changed to increasing satisfaction as they gained confidence in predicting results, on the basis of identification of three principles of concentric mastopexy to obtain breasts with areolas of a predictable size. Spear states:

First and most important, the outer concentric circle must be drawn so as not to exceed the original areola diameter by more than the inner concentric circle diameter. Second: the outer circle diameter be drawn not to exceed twice that of the inner circle, to prevent poor scarring or over flattening of the breast. Third: which allows prediction of the final areola size as the average of the diameters of the inner and outer concentric circles.

They believe these three principles allow excision of a maximum amount of areola and periareolar skin without the side effects of poor scars, dilated

Figure 2.11. Martins's transposition of flaps by a periareolar approach. The breast is divided transversely into two halves or hemispheres (*left*): an upper hemisphere, including the nipple-areolar unit, and a lower hemisphere serving to shape a glandular pad. This pad will act as a breast prosthesis, contributing to shaping and supporting the operated breast (*right*).

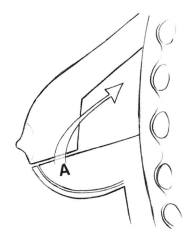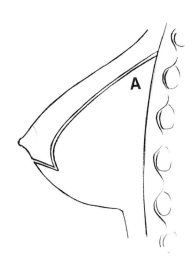

areola, or misshapen breasts. By applying these three principles, they believe one may correct a wide variety of deformities, producing more symmetrical, attractive breasts with areolas of predictable size. Spear believes the Benelli, Lejour, Marchac, and Wise techniques all have their indications.

Martins (Porto Alegre, Brazil) reported in 1991[36] a mammoplasty technique for medium hypertrophies and ptotic breasts employing transposition of flaps and a periareolar approach. The breast is divided transversely into two halves or hemispheres: an upper hemisphere, including the nipple-areolar unit, and a lower half, serving to shape a glandular pad. This pad will act as a breast prosthesis, contributing toward shaping and supporting the operated breast. Mammary reduction is obtained with partial, medial, and lateral resections of the lower half and starting from the base of the breast in the upper hemisphere.[37] The glandular pad is fashioned from the lower hemisphere of the breast that is usually resected in the other procedures. The nipple-areolar unit remains joined to the body of the gland and to the decorticated skin, since the resection in the upper half is accomplished from the base of the breast. He believes internal fibrosis will lend stability to the shape and avoid early postoperative recurrence of ptosis (Figure 2.11).

Robles (Buenos Aires) in 1992[38] modified some

technical aspects of Benelli's technique, improving the closure of the areola and eliminating the pleats. By using a straight needle and a continuous circular and deep suture, he closes the areola around a variable-size tube (called the "holder"). He described a new prosthesis, conical shaped to project the central area of the breast. He uses the technique for mastopexy in moderate ptosis and tuberous breasts. Areolar holders give symmetry of areolar diameter and sutures with straight needle prevent thick folding around the areola. The main disadvantage is that it cannot be used for hypertrophy and with poor skin laxity. There is a relative indication for small hypertrophy and severe ptosis by adding a vertical incision like the Lejour procedure.[39] He is pleased with the mastopexy obtained and says it is 30% of his mammary surgical practice. He is also pleased with the shape and breast projection obtained by his technique, especially with the use of the conic prosthesis.

Aboudib (Rio de Janeiro, Brazil) in 1994[40] based his personal periareolar technique on the principles of Bustos, without utilizing the supporting sheet. He developed some modifications in the treatment, resection, and rotation of the mammary tissue. Aboudib claims a limited result in cases of pure ptosis without gland resection. Severe ptosis and hypertrophies (over 600 g) are contraindicated. He uses the Pitanguy technique

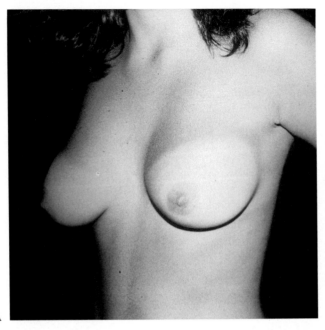
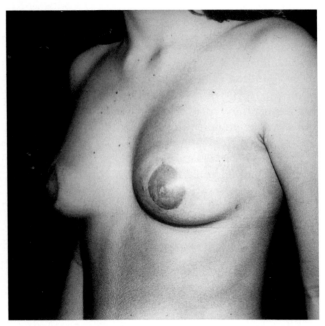

A

B

Figure 2.12. (A) Preoperative and **(B)** and postoperative result of Aboudib's approach to the Bustos technique, without the silicone sheet, in a patient with moderate hypertrophy and ptosis.

for those cases. Aboudib reports a minimum of complications. He uses the technique in 80% of his mammoplasty patients (Figure 2.12).

References

1. Davidson BA: Concentric circle operation for massive gynecomastia to excise the redundant skin. Plast Reconstr Surg 63(3):350–354, 1979.
2. Hinderer U: Una Nueva Técnica de Mastoplastias para Ptosis Ligeras. Presented at the VI Reunión Nacional de la Sociedad Española de Circurgía Plástica y Reparadora, Madrid, October 29–31, 1969.
3. Hinderer U: Una nueva técnica de mastoplastias para ptosis ligeras. Abstract published in *Noticias Médicas*, November 6, 1969, p. 28.
4. Joseph J: Zur Operation der Hypertrophischen Hangebrust. Dtsch Med Wochenschr 51:1003, 1925.
5. Noel MD: Methode Noel in der Modifikation von Cesary. Austrian Bull Sci Med 5, 1927.
6. Hinderer U: Plastia mamaria modelante de dermopexia superficial y retromamaria. Rev Esp Cir Plást 5(1):65, 1972.
7. Hinderer U: Development of concepts in reduction mammaplasty and ptosis. In: *Aesthetic Surgery of the Breast*. Georgiade NG, Georgiade GS, Riefkohl R (Eds.). W. B. Saunders Co., Philadelphia, 1990, pp. 565–603.
8. Andrews JM, Yshizuki MMA, Martins DMSF, Ramos RR: An areolar approach to reduction mammaplasty. Br J Plast Surg 28:166–170, 1975.
9. Arié G: Una nueva técnica de mastoplastia. Rev Latinoamericana Cir Plast 3:23, 1957.
10. Bartels RJ, Strickland DM, Douglas WM: A new mastopexy operation for mild or moderate ptosis. Plast Reconstr Surg 57(6):687–691, 1976.
11. Erol OO, Spira M: A mastopexy technique for mild and moderate ptosis. Plast Reconstr Surg 65(5):603–609, 1980.
12. Erol OO: Erol's periareolar mastopexy for different types of mammary ptosis (mild, moderate, severe, hypoplastic). In: *Annals of the International Symposium on Recent Advances in Plastic Surgery—RAPS 92*, March 14–15, 1992. Toledo LA (Ed.). Estadão, São Paulo, Brazil, 1992, p. 103.
13. Felício Y, Penaforte LR, Cruz VTF: Mamoplastia redutora com incisão periareolar. In: *Anais da 1a Jornada Sul Bras de Cirurgia Plástica*. Março 1984, SBCP (Ed.), Forianópolis, p. 307–311.
14. Felício Y: Mamaplastia de reduccion con solo una cicatriz periareolar. Rev Iberolatinoamericana Cir Plást 12:245, 1986.
15. Felício Y: Periareolar reduction mammoplasty. Plast Reconstr Surg 88(5):789, 1991.
16. Bustos RA, Loureiro LEK, Thame CC: Mamaplastia redutora de retalho lobular trilobulado de pedículo inferior por incisão periareolar. Trans XXIV Congr Bras Cir Plast, Gramado, APLUB, 1985, p. 484.
17. McKissock PK: Reduction mammaplasty with a vertical dermal flap. Plast Reconstr Surg 49:245, 1972.
18. Jurado J: Plasticas mamárias de redução baseadas em retalho dérmico vertical monopediculado. In: *Anais do XII Cong Bras de Cir Plast*. EMMA, 1976, p. 29.
19. Bustos RA: Periareolar mammoplasty with silicone supporting lamina. Plast Reconstr Surg 89(4):646, 1992.
20. Bustos RA: Personal communication, 1994.

21. Toledo LS, Matsudo PKR: Mammoplasty using liposuction and periareolar incision. In: *Abstracts Book of the IXth Congress of ISAPS*. New York, October 11–14, 1987, p. 35.
22. Toledo LS, Matsudo PKR: Mammoplasty using liposuction and periareolar incision. Aesth Plast Surg 13(1):9, 1989.
23. Toledo LS: Periareolar mammoplasty with syringe liposuction. In: *Annals of the International Symposium on Recent Advances in Plastic Surgery—RAPS 89*, March 3–5, 1989. Toledo LA (Ed.). Estadão, São Paulo, Brazil, 1989, p. 256.
24. Toledo LS: Mammoplasty using syringe liposuction and periareolar incision—a four year experience. In: *Annals of the IInd International Symposium on Recent Advances in Plastic Surgery—RAPS 90*, March 28–30, 1990. Toledo LS, Pinto EBS (Eds.). Marques Saraiva, São Paulo, Brazil, 1990, p. 127.
25. Peled IJ, Zagher U, Wexler MR: Purse string suture for reduction and closure of skin defects. Ann Plast Surg 14:465, 1985.
26. Benelli L: Technique de plastie mammaire le round block. Rev Fr Chir Esth 13(50):7, 1988.
27. Benelli L: A new periareolar mammaplasty: The "round block" technique. Aesth Plast Surg 14(2):93, 1990.
28. Wilkinson TS: The double Benelli stitch. Tech Forum 15(4):2, 1991.
29. Wilkinson TS: Principles of circumareolar mastopexy, as applied to breast repair and reconstruction. In: *Annals of the International Symposium on Recent Advances in Plastic Surgery—RAPS 92*, March 14–15, 1992. Toledo LS (Ed.). Estadão, São Paulo, Brazil, 1992, p. 129.
30. Hinderer U: Mammaplasty with a periareolar scar: Historical evolution and actual state. In: *Transactions of the Xth Congress of the IPRS* (Madrid), Vol. II. Elsevier Science Publishers, New York, 1992, pp. 569–571.
31. Ersek RA, Ersek SL: Circular cinching stitch. Plast Reconstr Surg 88(2):350, 1991.
32. Goes JCS: Periareolar mammaplasty: Double skin technique. Rev Bras Cir Plast 4(23):55, 1989.
33. Ribeiro L: *Cirurgia Plástica da Mama*. Medsi, Rio de Janeiro, 1989, pp. 185–266.
34. Spear SL, Kassan M, Little JW: Guidelines in concentric mastopexy. Plast Reconstr Surg 85(6):961, 1990.
35. Spear SL: Personal communication, 1994.
36. Martins PDE: Periareolar mammaplasty with flap transposition. Rev Bras Cir Plast 6(2):1, 1991.
37. Martins PDE: Periareolar mammaplasty—a personal technique. In: *Annals of the International Symposium on Recent Advances in Plastic Surgery—RAPS 92*, March 14–15, 1992. Toledo LS (Ed.). Estadão São Paulo, Brazil, 1992, p. 196.
38. Robles J: "Round block" technique—aportes técnicos personales. Rev Argent Cir Plást 2(1):57–65, 1992.
39. Lejour M, Abboud M, Declety A, Kertesz P: Reduction of mammoplasty scars: From a short infra-mammary scar to a vertical scar. Ann Chir Plast Esthét 35(5):369, 1990.
40. Aboudib JH: Mamoplastia Periareolar. In: *Atualização em Cirurgia Plástica Estética*, Robe, SBCPER, Regional S.P. (Ed.). 1994, pp 309–313.

Technical Points in Circumareolar Surgery: Deepithelialization

Tolbert S. Wilkinson

Owing to the increasing popularity of the circumareolar technique for a variety of problems, I was asked to chair a panel at the 1994 annual meeting of the American Society for Aesthetic Plastic Surgery. It is evident that a number of surgeons take moderately different approaches to the technique, beginning with Ulrich Hinderer, and continuing through the excellent video tape in 1993 by Larry Schlesinger. The only consensus is that the deepithelialized circle has been reduced by all authors and that a variety of methods are used to reduce tension to avoid spreading of the areola. The only radical departure is that of Cardoso de Castro, who has resumed the once discredited approach of circumferential freeing of skin from the breast and removing the wedge of tissue for reduction on the superior aspect. Complete exposure of the mound is used, so that circumferential tacking sutures may be employed to "fix the gland" at a higher position. American surgeons should be wary of this approach, although it seems to work well in his hands. This chapter contains an overview of technical maneuvers that are in wider use and those that have been contributed by a number of authors.

Technical Points in Circumareolar Breast Surgery

Standard mastopexy and breast reduction surgeries are fairly "cut and dried." When the markings are made, the surgeon simply follows the dotted lines and joins the marked points, and final adjustment is a relatively minor procedure. The circumareolar procedure, however, is more of a "hands-on" operation from start to finish.

In the circumareolar procedure, the technical maneuvers that we discuss in greater detail in subsequent chapters are extremely important in preventing or diminishing the incidence of the annoying complications that are unique to this procedure and that are common to all breast reductions, mastopexies, and internal repair surgeries.

When Louis Benelli first presented his "round block" technique and emphasized circle tension-relieving sutures, which were anchored to a deepithelialized bed of graft tissue, we had been undeterred by the complication of "severe areolar spreading." Multiple advancing sutures had diminished this complication but it still occurred

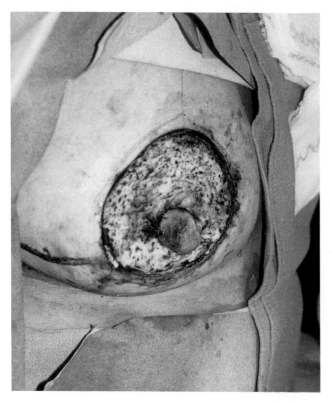

Figure 3.1. Complete preparation of the deepithelialized bed in circumareolar breast surgery.

with too great a frequency. As Gruber pointed out, there is a greater incidence of areolar spreading when an augmentation prosthesis is added.

My personal technique for the circle suture is to use a second "Benelli" suture of absorbable material that is closer to the areolar edge, thus minimizing the problem if the suture "spits" or becomes contaminated. As shown in Figure 3.1, the deepithelialized bed has been completely prepared before the skin is reflected. When the skin and subcutaneous fat are reflected, one may begin the heart of the procedure, which is to create the internal mound in breast reduction (by excision), in mastopexy (by infolding), or in repair of the overstretched breast (by left-to-right reinforcement).

Because earlier publications showed flattened and "pancake"-appearing breasts, with areolae set at a lower position, we discuss here the elevation of the areola by wedge excision, as proposed by Luiz Toledo. My modification of this is a triangular excision with the points of the triangle at the upper edge of the areola and the midline marking. Closure of this triangle sets the nipple at a higher position. One can then

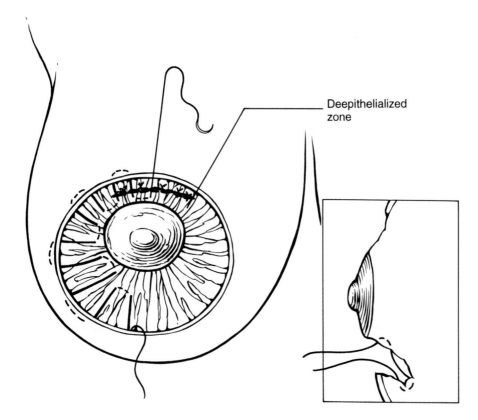

Deepithelialized zone

Figure 3.2. Placement of the first advancement suture, in the deep dermis of the breast skin, preparatory to raising the areola.

Figure 3.3. The second phase in elevating the areola: dimpling of the skin occurs as the suture is tied.

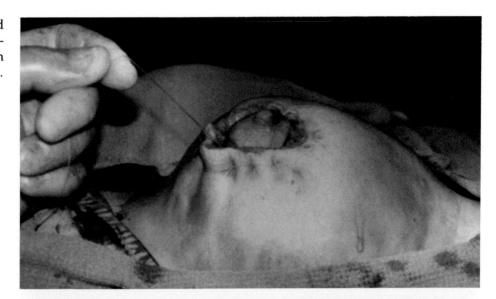

Figure 3.4. The third phase in elevation of the areola: after the sutures have been placed the skin and areolar edge touch, without pulling.

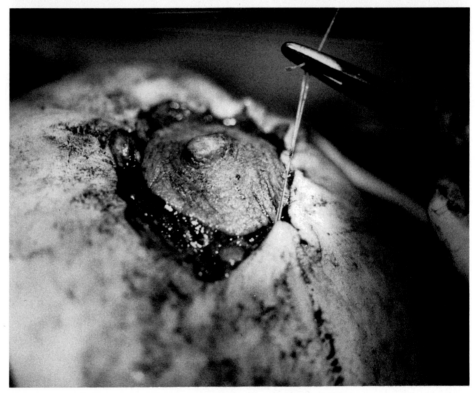

proceed to advance the skin to touch but not pull on the areolar edge. As shown in Figure 3.2, the first advancing suture is placed at a distance from the areolar skin edge and 1 cm or more underneath the breast skin. Locked into the deep dermis of the breast skin and the deepithelialized circle, this suture is advanced upward to bring the skin edges into apposition. Dimpling of the skin from the deep dermal bites is evident as the suture is tied (Figure 3.3). This suture is nonabsorbable, and therefore the initial knotting must be placed at a much deeper position to avoid surface contamination. When it is successfully placed, the skin edges will touch, when they are not retracted, by the natural elasticity of the breast tissue (Figure 3.4).

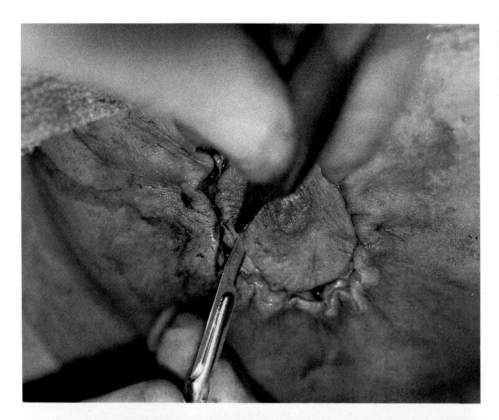

Figure 3.5. Everting the skin edges, by undercutting, stabilizes the nipple-areolar complex and enhances blood supply.

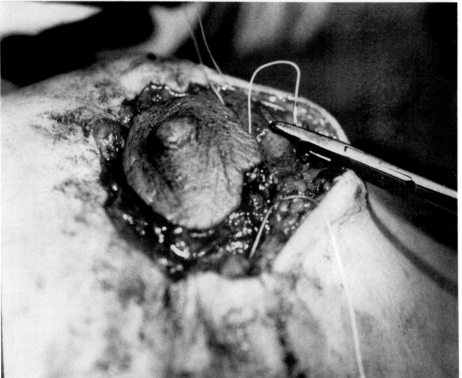

Figure 3.6. Placement of the second Benelli suture in circumareolar surgery.

In my technique, I do not undermine the skin over the upper third of the deepithelialized circle, to ensure a better blood supply and stability of the nipple-areolar complex. It is helpful, however, to undercut the skin edges so that they will evert (Figure 3.5).

The most important suture in circumareolar surgery is the second Benelli suture, which is absorbable. I prefer a Dexon 2-0 for this suture and a Mersilene 2-0 for the more distant suture, which is in a more protected position. The initial knot is also buried as far as possible from the surface (Figure 3.6). As the suture passes in a clockwise manner, tissue bites are made in the superficial dermis just beneath the skin edge of the breast skin, and into the dermis just below the edge of the areola (Figures 3.7 and 3.8). At the completion of the circular suture, the skin edges should be everted and touching, and the knot can then be buried by joining it to the original suture end, which has been left long for this purpose.

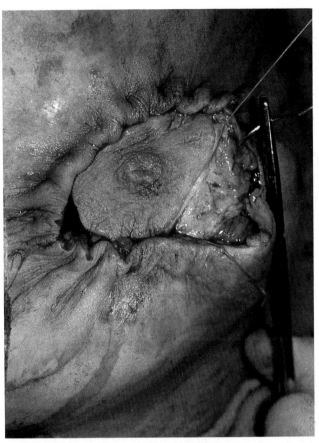

Figure 3.7. As the second Benelli suture is placed, the superficial dermis and dermis below the areolar edge are joined.

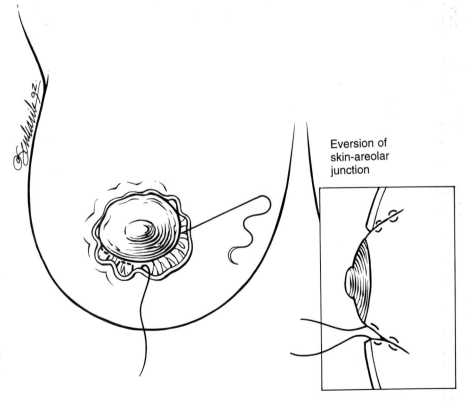

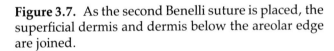

Eversion of
skin-areolar
junction

Figure 3.8. A diagram of the placement of the second Benelli suture.

On occasion, one may need Nylon 6-0 tacking sutures to correct any gapping that may occur.

The distant nonabsorbable suture relieves the tension on the second absorbable suture, which then brings the edges into approximation. Later, expansion of the areola, which has been reduced to 3.8 cm in most cases, obliterates the infolding at the edges.

Reducing the Internal Mound Distance

As shown in Chapters 8 and 9, and particularly in Figure 2 in Chapter 10 on breast repair, many patients have an excess amount of soft tissue between the new areola and the old inframammary fold. When the infolding procedure was first described by Erol (see Chapter 2), he emphasized setting the inframammary fold at a higher position. In many patients, this requires removal of the lower soft tissue to reduce the length of the internal mound to 6 cm. We suggest that it is not necessary to deepithelialize a circle that leaves only a 6-cm amount of skin, because the lower skin will retract, and it will also set into the space left by elevation of the inframammary fold if this is required. Setting the inframammary fold is technically difficult as well. I place the central suture into the fascia of the pectoralis muscle first, and then join to this the two limbs of the breast tissue that has been divided for entry into a breast prosthesis pocket in breast repair, or the edges that are exposed by resection or infolding in mastopexy and reduction. Once this primary suture has been set at the new position, additional sutures are placed laterally to ensure the rounding of the internal mound.

Contrast this repositioning of the nipple-areolar complex and skin advancement with the techniques that we employ in standard mastopexy. Because skin has been removed in the inverted "T" or "anchor," the new nipple-areolar complex can be secured in a superior position quite readily. In our early series of circumareolar mastopexies (Figures 3.9 and 3.10) we used a similar form of multilayered advancement, which did not control areolar expansion as well. We also brought skin inward from all quadrants, which

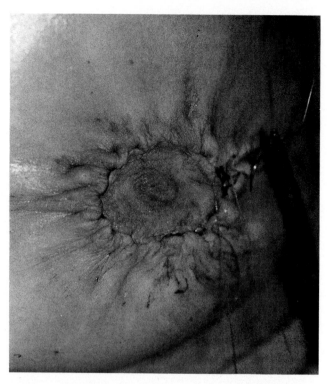

Figure 3.9. An early example of circumareolar mastopexy, in which a similar form of multilayered advancement was used.

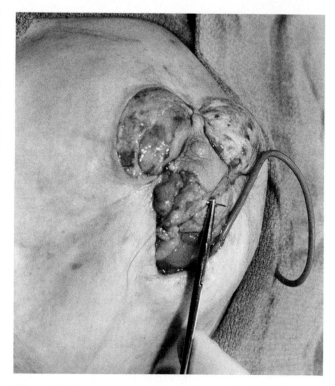

Figure 3.10.

frequently left the areola at a position lower than desired. As discussed by Drs. Aiache and Toledo, when marking the new nipple-areolar position, one should take measures to make certain that it remains at that level.

Infolding Technique

In performing a mastopexy on larger breasts, in which the areolar diameter must be reduced and the areola must be elevated, a wider lateral undermining is necessary, as shown in Figure 3.11. Prior to elevating the areola with the wedge excision, the hemostat is used to grasp the tissue to be infolded and it is held in its new elevated position until a #1 Vicryl suture has been tied down.

Figure 3.12 shows a completion of the basket weave infolding procedure. The areola has been moved to its new position and the subcutaneous mound has been created.

Scar Reduction

Obtaining a smooth, flat scar is one of our goals. Undermining the surrounding skin with a scalpel, both the areolar and breast skin, would have prevented the white zone from being as obvious (Figure 3.13). The second Benelli stitch everts the skin edges so that flattening occurs without widening. Undermining with a few passes of the scalpel blade does not compromise blood supply, but does ensure true and adequate skin edge eversion. I allow this eversion, which may need a few Nylon 6-0 tacking sutures for gaps (Figure 3.14), to remain unsupported until there is adhesion. Skin tapes of the mesh or strip type might force a "roll in" or inversion of these edges if used in the operating room. One additional factor is the inevitable oozing of tissue fluids and local anesthetic solutions between the edges. The surgeon accustomed to closing the areola in standard T-scar surgeries does not see this. In these cases, I use half-buried mattress sutures. In the circumareolar cases one does not sew breast skin

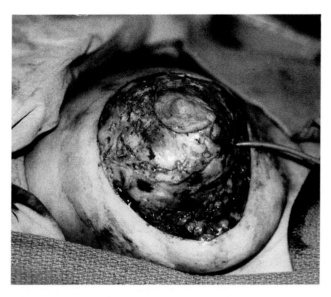

Figure 3.11. Wider lateral undermining is necessary when performing a mastopexy on larger breasts.

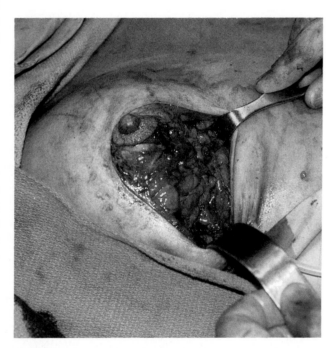

Figure 3.12. Completion of the basket weave infolding procedure.

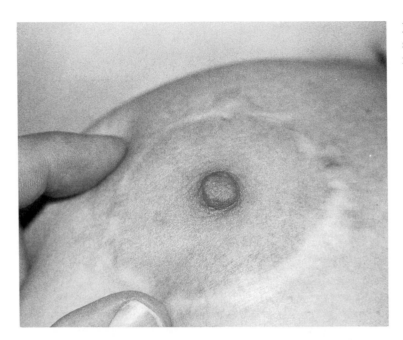

Figure 3.13. A fairly large white zone of scarring that could have been prevented by more adequate skin edge eversion.

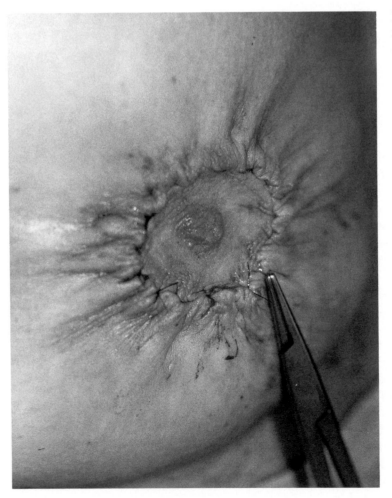

Figure 3.14. Application of Nylon 6-0 tacking suture to close a gap between areolar and breast skin.

to areolar skin. Fluid ooze between the everted edges would be trapped under the skin, causing maceration.

Postoperative Support

In all categories of circumareolar breast surgery (reduction, mastopexy, and repair and reshaping following implant removal) postoperative support of the soft tissue is essential. This promotes shrinkage of the reflected skin and protects internal suture integrity. Support of the skin incision is necessary as well. Because of the unique closure that I employ, with the skin edges everted and touching but not sutured, there is inevitably drainage between the skin edges. Therefore, tape supports (Steri-Strip type) are not applied until the second or third postoperative day. We have also used mesh tape, which will immobilize a 4-cm^2 area of skin while still allowing drainage between the expanded parts of the tape.

At the end of 7 days it is appropriate to further reinforce the areola with 1-in. paper tape, which is then coated with a sealant such as collodion. This allows the patient to bathe in her brassiere without the danger of water contamination of the incision. By the end of 14 days, patients are allowed to bathe in a tub and to remove the brassiere as long as they are recumbent.

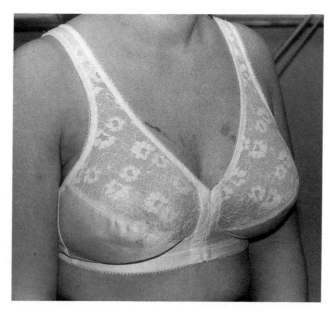

Figure 3.15. A front-hook, heavy support brassiere.

The selection of brassieres is important as well. Brassieres are used as a fixed support for the lower half of the breasts beginning 24 h after surgery and drain removal. Figure 3.15 shows the front-hook, heavy support brassiere that we supply to our patients. Patients certainly do not like shopping for brassieres and have no idea what "support" means. Our practice is to supply each patient with two postoperative brassieres, and a supply of skin creams that keep the skin comfort-

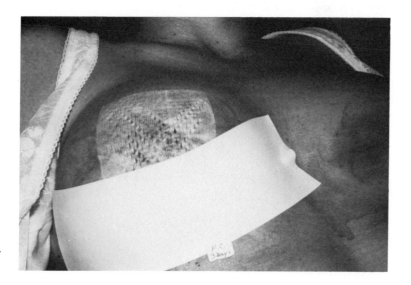

Figure 3.16. Elastic skin tape used to support the lower half of the breast.

able.* Our patients are allowed to open the brassiere at intervals for bathing purposes and to apply these lotions, particularly to areas where the strap of the brassiere circles the chest. By keeping the skin soothed and comfortable, patients are more likely to comply with our directives. In the larger breast reductions, constant wearing of the brassiere is required for 6 weeks and then intermittently and at night thereafter. For the small mastopexies or repair, we can usually change to a "softer," more elastic version of the front-hook support brassiere. Both of these brassieres are furnished to us by Medical Cosmetic Services and are given to the patients. The cost is part of the surgical fee.

For the larger reductions it is often helpful to use elastic skin tapes to support the lower half of the breast, particularly between the second and seventh day (Figure 3.16). These tapes will cause too much skin irritation if they are continued for a longer period of time but they do apply elastic pressure as well as support that is independent of the brassiere.

After 6 weeks, our patients visit the brassiere boutique in our clinic to select brassieres that are less supportive and more feminine. These are supplied for patient purchase as a convenience. Office personnel assist in brassiere fitting so that support is maintained, but not to the degree required in the early phases of recovery.

---

*Medical Cosmetic Services, 1901 Babcock Road, #201, San Antonio, Texas 78229.

The Circular Suture Technique, Markings, Skin Flaps, and Postsurgical Dressings

Introduction

Tolbert S. Wilkinson

Many of the innovations that were contributed by independent technical experimentation and change are now incorporated into the circumareolar procedure. For all categories of patients, as discussed in Chapter 1, the original approach to circumareolar surgery was to excise an appropriate circle of skin and subcutaneous tissue and then to advance breast skin from all sides toward the center. Not only did this leave the nipple in a lower position and make its position somewhat unpredictable during the healing phase, but the advancement sutures contributed to areolar enlargement. The addition of a deepithelialized ring provides a firm and stable floor onto which the advanced skin may attach, and a nonsliding area at some distance from the areolar skin edge in which to attach advancing sutures. Each of us uses slightly different techniques and different suture materials, but the principles are the same.

The Circular Suture Technique

Adrien Aiache

It was the experience of plastic surgeons that if a "doughnut" excision was performed on the breast, it often developed a secondary deformity consisting of the extreme enlargement of the areola, sometimes to the size of the original doughnut outer border and often associated with scar widening, making the result even more unsightly.

This problem has been the main reason for the limited popularity of the technique of periareolar mastopexy: the gradually enlarging areola marred the initially good results. To combat this effect, Benelli developed his "round block" idea. Basically, it consists of fixing the circumference of the areola and maintaining it with a nonabsorbable suture placed in the deep dermis.

Many discussions have been generated concerning this particular suture. Many attempts have been made to improve its effect on the skin and prevent secondary problems such as suture rejection or infection and eventually unilateral breakage, ending in unevenly sized areolas. This round block stitch is woven deeply in the dermis in exactly measured bites, allowing a symmetrical pleating of the skin around the block. It is placed deeply because it only secures the circumference of the areola, without any attempt at closing the wound. This suture must be placed away from the areas of the skin to be closed in layers. It is preferable to free the superior area of skin flap in obtaining a complete circular skin flap of the breast mound, in order to allow even, symmetrical pleating of the skin edges around the areola. This simple and original maneuver is the most important in assuring a stable areola. As mentioned in Chapter 3, the circular suture should allow the muscular areola to lay flat without stretching or bunching—the former responsible for postoperative paralysis of the areolar muscle and the latter causing a "Snoopy" deformity of the areola. If necessary, the skin should be free from the deep suture for proper and flat approximation to the areola during closure (Figure 4.1).

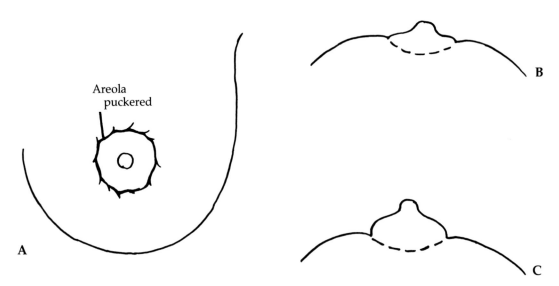

Figure 4.1. Schematic drawings of circumareolar scarring. **(A)** Starburst effect of the scar obtained by suturing a larger skin circle to a smaller one. This scar eventually improves in most cases. **(B)** Problems of scar inversion with retraction of the whole areola, sometimes obtained inadvertently by this technique. **(C)** Other problems sometimes secondary to the tightening effect of the unyielding scar, pushing out the areola in a "Snoopy"-type deformity.

Technical Points to Circumareolar Breast Surgery: Markings and Skin Flaps

Tolbert S. Wilkinson

As is emphasized repeatedly throughout this book, markings on the skin are not as important as the creation of the subcutaneous breast shape. Nevertheless, if an excess of skin is left in place, we cannot expect sufficient shrinkage to the new subcutaneous cone. On the other hand, the larger the circle of skin that is removed or deepithelialized, the more likely there is to be long-term wrinkling in the closure, and the greater the possibility that the surgeon will choose a "lollipop" vertical midline excision. In this book we assume that patient selection precludes the lollipop excision, and will demonstrate to you the technical maneuvers that virtually eliminate areolar spread and reduce the length of time in which the circumferential rippling is visible. In my technique, undermining is limited to the lower half or two thirds of the breast. Other authors have no hesitation in undermining all of the breast skin, which diminishes blood supply. With the fixation techniques now available for the new nipple-areolar complex, and the possibility

of compromised blood supply in the larger patient, I believe superior undermining to be unnecessary, as well as adding an element of risk.

Markings

There are many formulas for marking; they range from the more complex ones described by Scott Spear to the simplest. My approach to the markings is a simple one.

The first marking, as shown in Figure 4.2, is the ideal position for the top of the newly reduced areola. The measurements are made as for standard reductions or mastopexies and then visually adjusted. Notice the change in the line on the left breast. The second marking is from the edge of the new areola to the inframammary fold. In our original series we made a wider skin excision in this area so that we would leave the ideal 5 to 6 cm. Notice in Figure 4.3 that this distance has

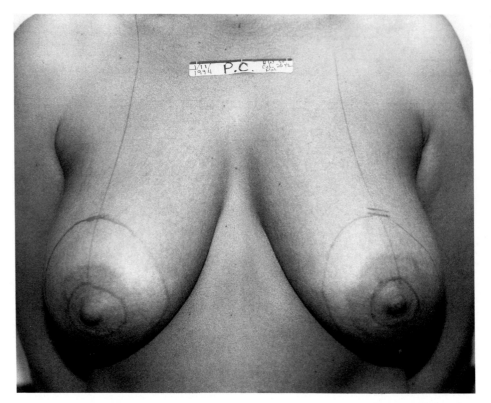

Figure 4.2. Initial markings for ideal positions for the tops of the reduced areolae, and from the edge of the new areola to the inframammary fold.

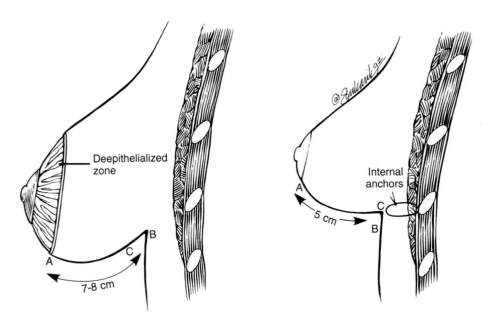

Figure 4.3. Point A, edge of breast skin; point B, old inframammary fold; point C, new inframammary fold.

been left between 7 and 8 cm, because contracture will reduce the length of this skin. This is the skin that is reflected during the procedure. Also note that if a new inframammary fold is selected, the excess skin will be taken up by filling this void. The old inframammary fold (Figure 4.3, point B) is now covered by breast skin (Figure 4.3, point C).

The other important change is that the internal cone shape, which is set at an ideal distance, is more important than the skin that covers it. The skin of patients who are "good" candidates for circumareolar surgery will contract and contour to the new shape, much as the skin in the male neck will contour to a resutured and liposuctioned submental repair.

With these two markings in place, I simply estimate the amount of skin that must be removed laterally and medially. This varies from side to side (Figure 4.4A and B).

As is emphasized throughout this book, the most important maneuver is the creation of the subcutaneous breast mound. One does not wish to leave too much lateral and medial skin; on the other hand, the smaller the deepithelialized circle the less likely it is that it will show folding as a result of skin advancement, 3 and 6 months after surgery.

How Much Should You Leave on the Skin Flap?

Since the circumareolar procedure is so technically dependent, and we count on skin shrinkage, the question of how much fat to leave on the reflected skin is of greater importance in this procedure than in others. If the skin is reflected at the deep dermis level, the blood supply is more tenuous and the breast is more likely to suffer damage from pressure or trauma.

One such case, which occurred in 1981, was the subject of a lawsuit. She was the only patient in

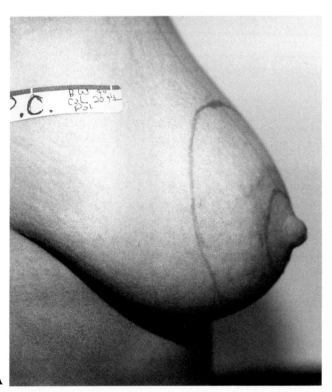
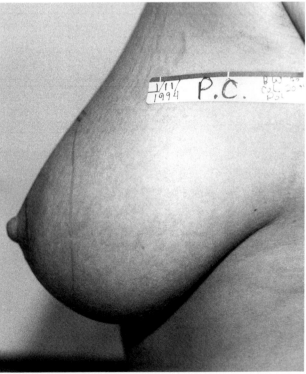

A   **B**

Figure 4.4. Final markings: Amount of skin to be removed laterally and medially. Shown here is a comparison of markings on patient P.C.'s left breast **(A)** and right breast **(B)**. Note they are not identical.

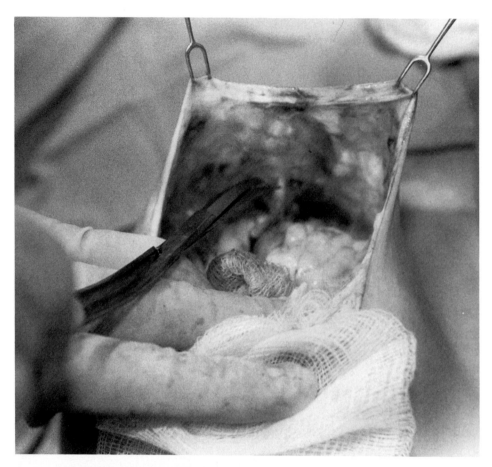

Figure 4.5. Dissection, using the curved facelift scissor, above the breast parenchyma.

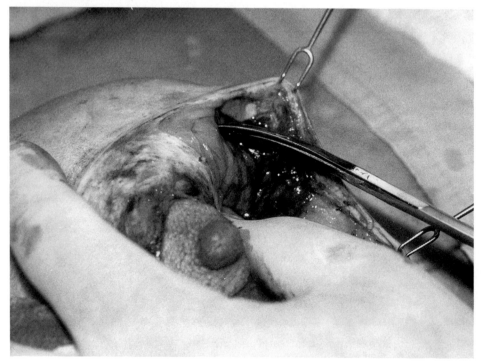

Figure 4.6. Further dissection using the curved facelift scissor—curvature of the scissor makes it easier to follow the breast wall.

whom I have lost skin in the area between the nipple and the inframammary fold. This patient suffered a fall that not only injured her abdominoplasty, creating a seroma, but led to a 2-cm necrosis on one breast in the midportion between the areola and the inframammary fold.

The seroma may have been related to the use of the Shrudde curettage method, which preceded liposuction of the upper abdomen and limited abdominoplasty, or to trauma. The skin of the breast would likely have survived the trauma had a greater cushion been left in place to protect it from the stiffness of the underlying mattress sutures that infolded the breast.

As we have noted, the new design of the circumareolar deepithelialization leaves a greater amount of skin between the edge of the areola and the inframammary fold, not only because the fold will be repositioned at a higher position but because of shrinkage. The higher repositioning allows 2 to 3 cm of skin to fall against the chest wall and the shrinkage should account for the remainder. In Figure 4.5, you can see that a careful dissection has been carried out just above the thickness of the breast parenchyma. I use the curved facelift scissor (Wilkinson's facelift scissor; Snowden-Pencer, Atlanta, Georgia) because the flat blades and wide, blunt tips allow spreading dissection as well as cutting dissection. The curvature makes it easy to follow the breast wall, as shown in Figure 4.6. With two hooks suspending the skin and the operator's left hand holding the breast mass away, it is very easy to stay in the deep fatty plane.

One axiom is that it is far easier to trim away any excess fat left on the skin flap than it is to repair an area of exposed dermis. The thickness of the fat also gives a contour cushion that will hide any small surface irregularities in the subcutaneous breast cone.

Once the inframammary fold area has been reached, the spreading motion of the scissors exposes the pectoralis muscle. Dissection should be carried out laterally and medially until sufficient space is exposed for the infolding, splitting, or triangular resection.

Postsurgical Dressings

Tolbert S. Wilkinson

Because of the unique nature of the circumareolar mastopexy, dressings are of paramount importance. There is no skin brassiere to reinforce the internal sutures of a reduction or mastopexy or repair.

The patient in Figures 4.7 through 4.9 illustrates the phases in dressing changes following a circumareolar repair after breast prosthesis removal.

In circumareolar surgery protective padding dressings are used, but no tapes are applied across the areolar incisions and no skin tapes are used for support, in order to preserve blood supply and to allow free drainage of the lidocaine (Xylocaine) mixture and serum from around the areola. The patient in Figures 4.7 through 4.9 underwent liposuction, rhinoplasty, and breast reduction under ketamine-diazepam (Valium) "twilight" anesthesia in our clinic. Anesthesia is more easily obtained by the infusion technique, in which a small stab wound is made at the lateral inframammary fold and 500 cm^3 of 0.25% Xylocaine with epinephrine is infiltrated throughout the subcutaneous tissue under the breast and throughout the surrounding tissues, using a blunt 14-gauge instillation needle.

Twenty-four hours after surgery the patient is ready for tape reinforcement. The tape illustrated in Figure 4.7 is Mesh tape (3M Company). This square of tape, when it is expanded, immobilizes not only the areolar edges but the surrounding skin as well. The expanded openings allow free drainage. This tape is left in place for approximately 2 weeks. The patient is allowed to change dressings above it after 1 week.

After the third to fourth day, supporting stretched Micropore tape (3M Company) is applied to hold the skin in its new position in the elevated inframammary fold and against the internal repair (Figure 4.8). These tapes are left in place for 2 weeks.

Figure 4.9 shows a patient wearing a supportive brassiere. This front-hook brassiere is less heavily constructed than the one used in the first six weeks after surgery (Figure 3.15). At the end of 3 weeks, patients are allowed to remove the brassiere while bathing in a tub. At the end of 6 weeks, this stretchy, softer version of the front-hook support bra is employed, and after 10 weeks our clinic patients visit our "bra boutique" to select brassieres that will fit their new shape. At this point, it seems perfectly safe to allow them to

Figure 4.7. When it is expanded, Mesh tape (3M Company) immobilizes not only the areolar edges but the surrounding skin as well.

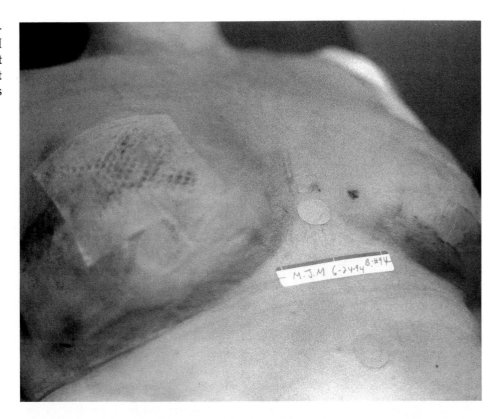

Figure 4.8. Supporting stretched Micropore tape (3M Company) is applied to hold the skin in its new position in the elevated inframammary fold and against the internal repair.

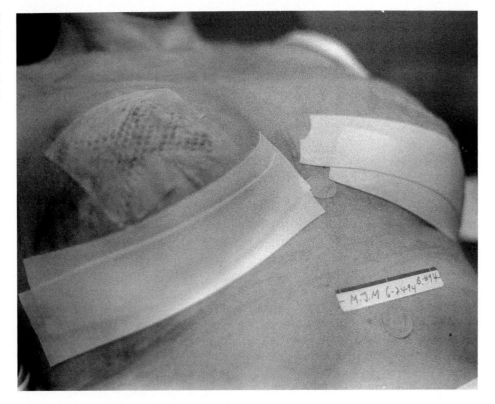

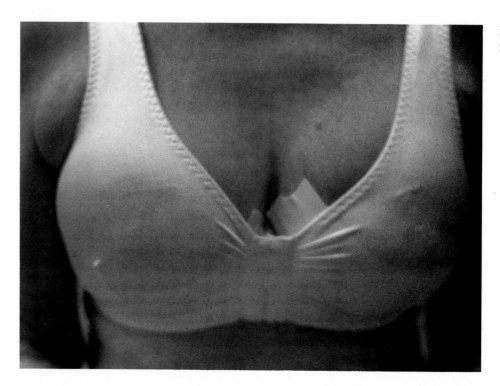

Figure 4.9. A patient wearing a supportive brassiere.

use underwire brassieres. Use of an underwire brassiere in the early healing phases would embarrass blood supply to the lower skin flap.

During this extended recovery time, patients are shown the use of skin creams and oils that reduce swelling and maintain skin comfort. This patient packet is provided for us by Medical Cosmetic Services (San Antonio, TX). By the end of 6 weeks, vigorous finger tip massage to "iron out" the folds is a safe maneuver and facilitates smoothing of the skin.

❖ 5 ❖

Role of Liposuction in Circumareolar Surgery

Tolbert S. Wilkinson and Luiz S. Toledo

Introduction

Tolbert S. Wilkinson

When the authors of this text gather for our annual teaching course on circumareolar surgery, we like to tease Luiz Toledo with the comment that was made when he gave a presentation many years ago on liposuction in breast reduction and mastopexy. He was told, "Son, we don't suction breasts in this country." Today, liposuction is an integral part of these procedures. The original fear that it would leave disturbing tracks and confuse radiologists has been put to rest. As noted in Chapter 1, and in case presentations by Alan Matarasso, Eugene Courtiss, and others, liposuction alone is the procedure of choice for certain secondary breast reductions and as a primary, less traumatic method of breast reduction in the elderly patient.

There is certainly no argument that liposuction may be used to adjust the volume of breasts in reduction surgeries or mastopexies. The only cautionary note is that in larger breasts in which major reductions are being performed, liposuction may embarrass blood supply should bleeding occur. This would be more of a concern with a younger, more vascular breast. Minor adjustments, however, are relatively risk free.

With good-quality breast skin that will shrink to a new shape, and the addition of liposuction for further adjustment, skin excision beyond the circle is unnecessary in all but the largest breasts. This is in disagreement with proponents of the vertical excision, commonly called the "lollipop" conversion, discussed in Chapter 6. Liposuction as a primary means of reduction does not address the formation of a lifted conical breast, or the reinforcement of the soft tissues from a flaccid state to a more stable state; nor does it address the removal of glandular tissue and repositioning and/or reduction of the areola. Therefore, liposuction as a primary means of reduction must be viewed as an appropriate procedure only for a small subgroup of individuals in whom the aesthetics are unimportant.

Luiz Toledo should be given the credit for popularizing the use of liposuction in moderate breast reductions and mastopexies. His experience is certainly extensive. I attribute this to the preferences of Brazilians for smaller, more compact breasts, as opposed to the American preference for expanded, augmented breasts!

The Role of Liposuction in Breast Reduction

Luiz S. Toledo

Plastic surgery techniques changed radically after the introduction of liposuction. Many existing concepts were reevaluated, the most significant being that it was no longer necessary to produce a large scar to alter the shape of the body. In the late 1970s dermolipectomies usually involved extensive scarring. The advent of liposuction made it possible for us to modify the body contour with minimal incisions, no skin resections, more natural results, and happier patients. Liposuction has seen many refinements, in technique and instruments. We prefer syringe liposuction; it is, in our hands, a much more gentle and precise method of fat removal, allowing us to treat more accurately small pair adiposities, such as the breasts.

We started performing breast liposuction in 1985, presented and published as an abstract for the first time in 1987,[1,2] and the detailed paper in 1989.[3] Initially we used the liposuction aspirator, and changed to disposable syringes in 1988.[4,5] Suction is used as an adjunct to mammoplasty, or as a means of its own to reduce the breast. Our method of breast reduction, a combination of liposuction and the periareolar incision, offers a good alternative procedure to correct asymmetries, and small to medium hypertrophies; to

reduce and perform the mastopexy, the mastopexy without reduction, or the mastopexy combined with augmentation using silicone prosthesis; all while removing little, or no skin at all. The fatty portion of the breast can be visualized by roentgenography[6] or by a computerized tomography (CT) scan. We can considerably reduce a fatty breast by syringe liposuction alone, using one or two cannula incisions (Figures 5.1 and 5.2). With superficial suction we provoke skin retraction, allowing us to treat older patients with more flaccid skin (Figure 5.3), patients that would not be indicated as good liposuction patients.

Until recently, most reduction mammoplasty techniques were based on the theory that skin removal was essential to obtain a successful result, although we know, by observing pregnant women, that skin tends to retract spontaneously. The development of tissue expanders is also based on this principle. Staub, Bzowski, and Vilain[7] showed in a series of 34 cases that juvenile mammary hypertrophy can be treated by performing glandular resections through an isolated inframammary incision, without skin excision, thus preventing secondary ptosis and stretch marks.

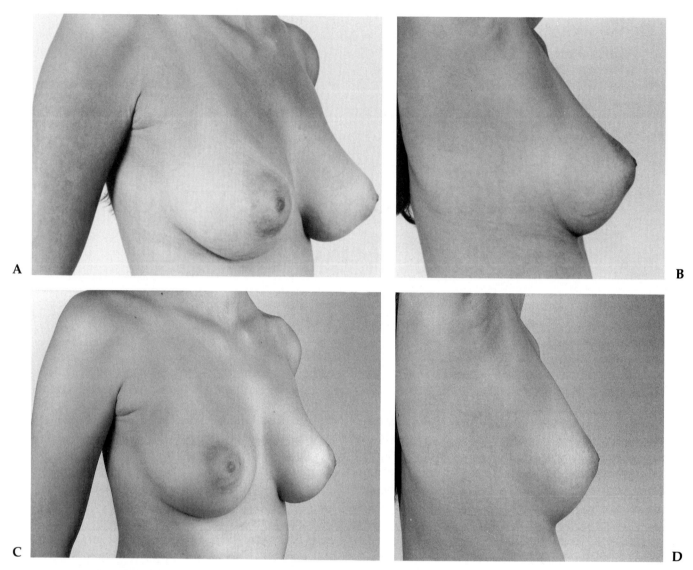

Figure 5.1. (A, B) Preoperative appearance of a 16-year-old patient before breast syringe liposuction. **(C, D)** Six months postoperative, with a good reduction in breast size and weight, correction of ptosis, and reduction of areolar diameter.

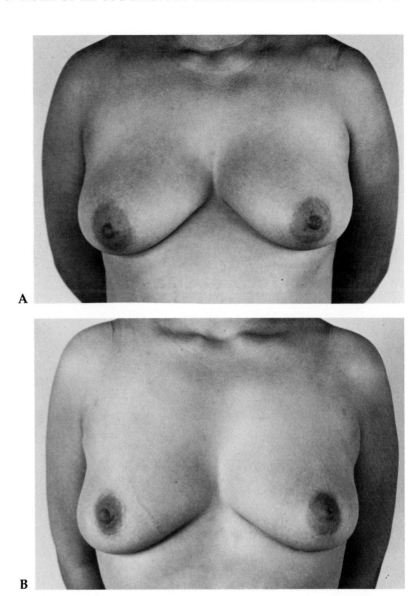

Figure 5.2. (A) Preoperative appearance of a 30-year-old patient before breast syringe liposuction. **(B)** One year postoperative, with a good reduction in breast size and weight, correction of ptosis, and reduction of areolar diameter. Patient also had suction in flanks and abdomen.

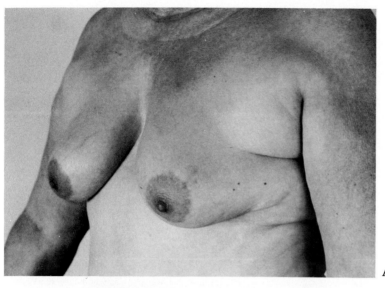

A

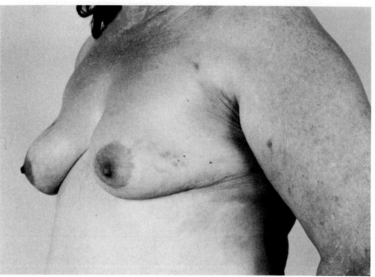

B

Figure 5.3. **(A)** Preoperative appearance of a 53-year-old patient, before breast syringe liposuction; this patient had submitted to reduction mammoplasty 20 years earlier. Her major complaint was of excess fat laterally and under the arms. **(B)** Six months postoperative, with a good skin retraction, improvement of ptosis, and reduction of areolar diameter.

We agree that suction should be the technique of choice for young patients with medium hypertrophies that have yet not reached full development of breasts, but need reduction before the process affects skin elasticity and before the breast weight provokes posture problems.

Anesthesia

Preoperative tests include a complete blood count, coagulation tests, and tests for glycemia and human immunodeficiency virus (HIV), plus a clinical evaluation and electrocardiogram (EKG).

For suction we use our local anesthesia formula,[7] a modification of Klein's tumescent technique,[9] even when associated with general anesthesia, high epidural, or local combined with intravenous (i.v.) sedation. The solution consists of 500 cm³ of Ringer's lactate, 20 cm³ of 2% lidocaine, 1 cm³ of adrenaline (1:1000), and 10 cm³ of 3% sodium bicarbonate.[10] Sodium bicarbonate eliminates the pain of injection of the anesthetic fluid.[11] We increased the lidocaine dose to treat regions closer to the skin. We keep the solution at room temperature. We do not believe cold solutions prevent bleeding for the necessary period of surgery and they are very uncomfortable to the patient. The formula helps to control bleeding. If we plan to remove up to 1 liter of fat we use only local anesthesia with oral sedation (midazolam, 15 mg) in ambulatory patients. When we combine suction and mastopexy we use a stronger solution for the skin (0.5% lidocaine with epinephrine [1:100,000 or 1:200,000]), in doses up to 500 mg.[12] In severe hypertrophies with suction and glandular resection, we combine local with high epidural or general anesthesia and a 12- to 24-hr hospital stay.

The maximum recommended dose of lidocaine hydrochloride with epinephrine is 7 mg/kg, with a total dosage of 500 mg.[13] As this is the limit amount of circulating drug, we can inject more solution subcutaneously safely (3550 mg of lidocaine, five to seven times over the traditional limit),[14] keeping a low drug level in the plasma. Not that we would need to inject all that amount of anesthesia for breast surgery, but it is good to know that we can if we have to. It is necessary to wait 15 min after the injection of the local anesthesia solution before start of suctioning.

Technique

We inject the anesthesia with a blunt, multiholed 2 or 3 mm-gauge needle. To perform breast liposculpture we use a 60-cm³ disposable syringe, connected to a 3, 4, or 5 mm-gauge, 20- to 35-cm-long cannula (Figure 5.4). We use cannulas with different tips, according to the case. We start with "pyramid" three-holed tip cannulas, and if there is some difficulty in suction we can use a more aggressive tip such as the Toledo dissector cannula, or the Becker cannula (Figure 5.5).

The cannula is inserted through an incision in the inframammary fold and through another in the axilla, for criss-crossing (Figure 5.6, right). We can reach the lateral chest wall, the axillary fold, the medial part of the breast, and the base of the mammary cone. We perform the glandular resection through a periareolar incision. We do not rely on skin to maintain the breast in place; the new shape is maintained by a combination of suction, gland resection, and secure mastopexy.

When there is no need for reduction we can perform mastopexy alone, through the periareolar incision. For medium hypertrophies we can reduce the breast by suction alone and perform the mastopexy (Figure 5.7). On large hypertrophies we have removed up to 1 kg of fat per breast, first suctioning up to 500 cm³ of fat on each side and then resecting the glandular tissue through the periareolar incision. If augmentation is desired we can improve the shape with suction and insert a silicone prosthesis after the mastopexy.

Dressings are very important to maintain the shape in the early postoperative days, while skin is retracting. We use Micropore tape dressings on the periareolar scar, covered by a gauze dressing, changed daily for 1 week. Suction drains stay for

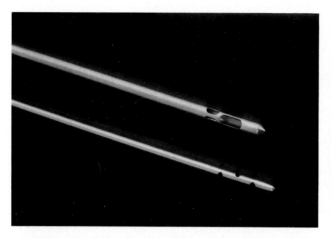

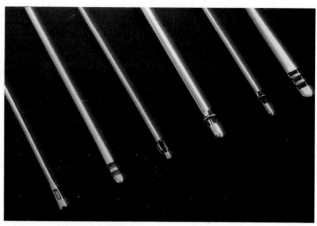

Figure 5.4. *Below:* A multiholed 3 mm-gauge blunt cannula for anesthesia injection. Slow injection of the formula is painless. *Above:* A 3.7 mm-gauge "pyramid" tip cannula used for syringe fat suction. (Both cannulas manufactured by The Tulip Company, San Diego, CA).

Figure 5.5. A collection of "aggressive" cannulas: From left: Toledo dissector cannula (Tulip Co.), two-holed flat rasping cannula (Grams Medical, Costa Mesa, CA), and four Becker cannulas (Wells Johnson, Tucson, AZ).

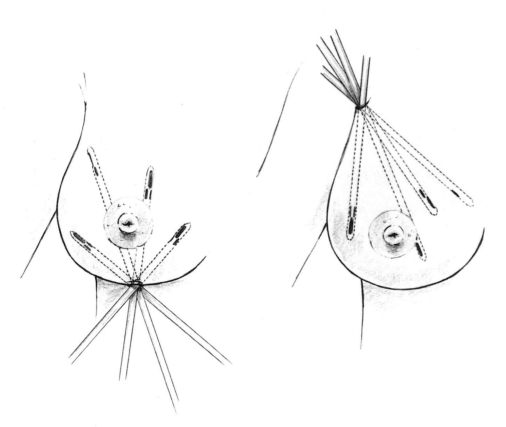

Figure 5.6. Cannula can be inserted through the submammary fold (left), and through the axilla (right), for "criss-crossing."

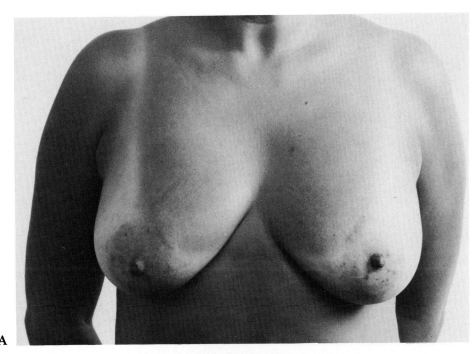

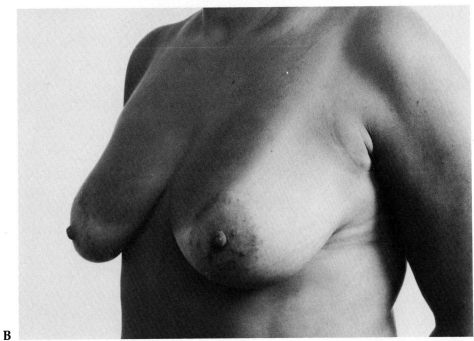

Figure 5.7. **(A–C)** Preoperative appearance of a 34-year-old patient before breast syringe liposuction combined with gland reduction. **(D–F)** Six months postoperative, with a good reduction of breast size and weight, correction of ptosis, and reduction of areolar diameter. Scar hypochromia can be corrected by tatooing.

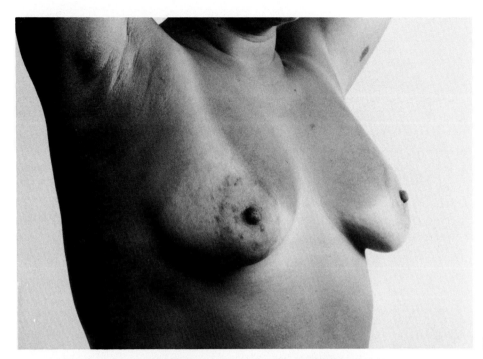

Figure 5.7C

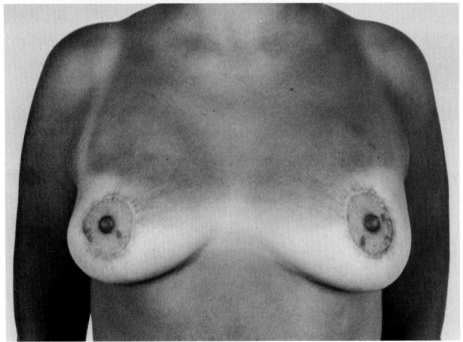

Figure 5.7D

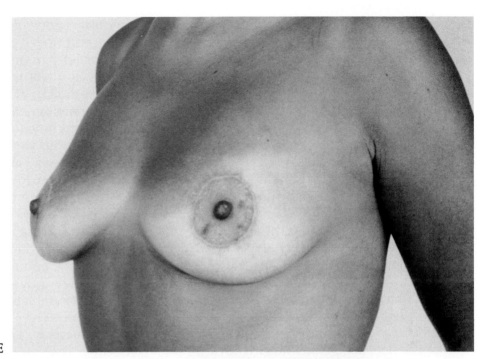

Figure 5.7E

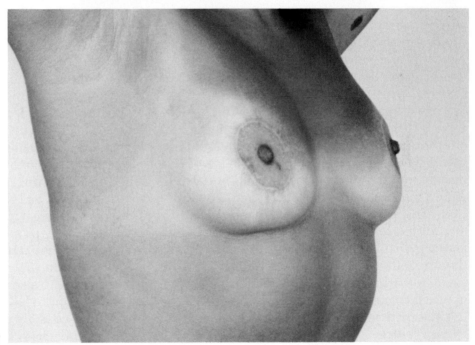

Figure 5.7F

5 to 7 days, or until the amount of fluid suctioned in 24 hr is around 50 cm³. An elastic brassiere should be worn constantly for 30 days.

Discussion

One of the main difficulties in the use of suction for breast reduction is that it is difficult to learn the technique. It is not something that can be measured, patterned, and schematized. There is an important component of "sculpturing" involved, as in any other surgery involving suction for body contouring.

Liposuction has been used since 1985 as an adjunct to breast reduction by Teimourian, Massac, and Weigering[15] and by Avelar[16] for breast reduction itself. Although it seems obvious that we can use liposuction only on fatty breasts, we have suctioned breast tissue. This we learned while treating gynecomastia. After suctioning the fat from the male breast, in some cases we were still not satisfied and we had to remove excess gland, causing an unnecessary areolar scar.

Some surgeons do not like to suction breasts; there is a theoretical concern that suction might affect breast function. In practice, however, surgeons have been using suction now for over a decade, not only for female breasts, but also in gynecomasties, with great success and few complications. Alterations in breast function are usually related to the condition of the breast before surgery, that is, recurrent mastitis or fibrocystic disease, rather than to the trauma of suction. The claim is that microcalcifications after breast surgery can be confused with the calcification of the in situ carcinoma, but all types of breast surgery, even a biopsy, can provoke calcification. For example, we did not diagnose any calcification in three of our patients, but in each we could palpate a small cyst that, after removal, was shown by a pathologist to be fat necrosis.

It is important to ask for a preoperative mammogram followed by another 6 months postoperatively, to evaluate the changes produced by the surgery. The objection that suctioning could induce calcifications of the breast is not a specific problem with this technique. It has been shown that reduction mammoplasty techniques can produce calcifications in the breasts even without suction. Mitnick, Roses, Harris, and Colen[17] studied mammograms of 152 patients after mammoplasty and noted calcifications in 37 patients. The calcifications were found to occur within the skin of the breast, mainly at a periareolar location. The ability to identify these benign calcifications further aids in reliably monitoring patients by mammography after reduction mammoplasty. Buhtz, Freitag, Berge, and Pohl[18] studied mammographic changes following reduction mammoplasty, and found that they can be relatively easily differentiated from malignant changes. Bilateral calcifications, they say, in most cases are caused by calcified fat necrosis.

Cruz, Guerrero, and Gonzalez[19] studied 100 consecutive cases of reduction mammoplasty. Of the group studied, only 1% showed atypical ductal hyperplasia and no cases of lobular carcinoma in situ or ductal carcinoma in situ were found. Fifty percent of the specimens showed simply fibrosis of the stroma dominating the gross and microscopic picture. The other pathological findings in descending order of frequency were cysts (30%), epithelial hyperplasia without atypia (6%), adenosis (5%), and apocrine metaplasia (5%). Clugston, Son-Hing, and MacFarlane[20] believe reduction mammoplasty may give rise to parenchymal scarring that may complicate subsequent clinical and radiological assessment of tumors. They propose preoperative mammography and state that biopsy may still be necessary to detect breast cancer after reduction mammoplasty. Perras[21] also recommends preoperative mammography. He has performed mammography before cosmetic surgery of the breast in a series of 1149 cases from 1973 to 1989, and has detected breast cancer in 34 cases. Cathcart and Hagerty[22] have pointed out that the lifetime breast cancer risk in the female population is 1 in 10. As this group of patients ages, it is obvious that surgeons will encounter carcinoma of the breast more frequently and that we must be prepared to face this fact.

Several surgeons use liposuction as an adjunct

to breast surgery. Pinnella[23] uses the liposuction cannula to create an inframammary crease, in the same way prescribed by Illouz to create a gluteal fold. Vinnik[24] uses suction lipoplasty to treat silicone-injected breasts. Drever[25] uses suction in breast reconstruction, "since the new breast is made of fat, we can change its size, enhance its shape, and sculpture it with a suction lipectomy cannula to make it look practically identical to the opposite, without compromising the vascularity of the flap." The breast may be accessed through the axilla, the areolar and inframammary areas, and through remote sites in the periumbilical area when other surgery is being performed. The breast may also be accessed when the flap is elevated during an abdominoplasty procedure. Erol[26] (Istanbul, Turkey), one of the pioneers in the periareolar technique, divides breasts into 11 groups and has a different approach for each group. He uses liposuction in two of them, for "moderate ptosis with very soft gland, consisting mainly of soft tissue and good skin quality" and "moderate breast ptosis with hypertrophic gland and good skin quality which needs reduction."

Matarasso and Courtiss[27] use suction lipectomy to reduce large breasts, as the sole technique in congenital asymmetry or in postreduction enlargement or asymmetry. Candidates for "suction alone" surgeries must fulfill two criteria: first, the nipple-areolar complex must be aesthetically well located; second, on physical examination their breast enlargement must be due primarily to fat. They use the technique not only in primary cases, but also in secondary ones if the patients fulfill these two criteria.

Samdal[28] relates one case of syringe liposculpture of the breasts followed by simple mastopexy on an outpatient basis. He believes an "ordinary reduction mammoplasty (Strombeck, McKissock) demands a relatively long anesthesia time and sometimes there is significant blood loss." After the aspiration, the skin was denuded according to the Strombeck pattern drawn before the operation.

Grazer[29] believes that, in the young patient, breast reduction by suction alone has many advantages over traditional techniques. He published a description of a patient who had breast implants and mastopexy, who some years later decided to change to smaller breast prostheses. Indeed, Grazer removed 300 cm^3 of breast tissue by suction, with a gratifying result.

Avelar and Illouz[16] say that as the balance between glandular and adipose tissue in the breast is altered after the fourth decade in life, with a reduction of gland and an increase of fat, it is possible to perform liposuction of the breast as a complement to reduction mammoplasty, in order to remove adipose tissue from the medial and axillary poles. They emphasize, however, that only fat, not glandular tissue, should be removed by suction. He also advocates pure suction for selected cases, that is, fatty breasts with no flaccidity or ptosis.

Illouz[30] points out that "we should make a distinction between the breasts themselves and the areas around the breast, like the anterolateral, the infra-mammary, lateral and the true axillary fat deposits. It may seem logical to reduce female breasts by aspiration, but it is illogical to think of reducing the size of a gland in this way."

When breast hypertrophy is associated with a significant degree of surrounding obesity and the breast appears to have extensions medially, laterally, or superiorly, owing to the excess of fat in these areas, Aiache[31] believes that "suction lipoplasty is particularly helpful in cases of reduction mammoplasty, by removing the excess fat present medially, laterally, and superiorly, and that liposuction often improves the actual shape of the breast, with less bleeding than when the dissection is performed." Also, Aiache believes that suction helps to improve the "dog ear" that is often present after the inverted T technique, allowing for a shorter scar. Aiache does not perform glandular removal by suction itself, advocating that it should be performed by whatever technique of reduction mammoplasty is preferred by the surgeon.

But Stark, Gramdel, and Spilker[32] use liposuction either alone or combined with resection for the correction of male and female breast deformities, and aspirate glandular tissue as well. The majority of the 32 patients in their study were treated for gynecomastia (69%). Other indications were Madelung's disease, gender dysphoria, asymmetry, hypertrophy, and postburn and postreconstruction deformities. In 54% of the gynecomastia cases, suction alone gave a satisfactory result. Only one male patient, treated by suction, needed an incision other than the periareolar. Thirteen aspirates from gynecomastias and three glands resected secondarily after suction were examined histologically. All aspirates included glandular tissue. They conclude that breast tissue is accessible to the suction cannula, and that this is a valuable tool for correcting gynecomastia and for use in many aesthetic procedures on the breasts of female patients.

References

1. Toledo LS, Matsudo PKR: Mammoplasty Using Liposuction and the Periareolar Incision. Presented at the IXth Congress of the International Society for Aesthetic Plastic Surgery, New York, October 11–14, 1987.
2. Toledo LS, Matsudo PKR: Mammoplasty using liposuction and the periareolar incision. In: *Abstract Book of the IXth International Congress of ISAPS.* New York, 1987, p. 35.
3. Toledo LS: Periareolar mammoplasty with syringe liposuction. In: *Annals of the International Symposium on Recent Advances in Plastic Surgery—RAPS 89,* March 3–5, 1989. Toledo LS (Ed.), Estadão, São Paulo, Brazil, 1989, p. 256.
4. Fournier P: *Liposculpture—Ma Technique.* Arnette, Paris, 1989.
5. Toledo LS, Matsudo PKR: Mammoplasty using liposuction and the periareolar incision. Aesth Plast Surg 13(1):9–13, 1989.
6. Douglas KP, et al.: Roentgenographic evaluation of the augmented breast. South Med J 84(1):49, 1991.
7. Staub S, Bzowski, A, Vilain R: Hypertrophie mammaire juvènile. Traitement chirurgical prècoce [Juvenile mammary hypertrophy. Early surgical treatment]. Ann Chir Plast Esthet 34(3):269, 1989.
8. Toledo LS: Superficial syringe liposculpture. In: *Annals of the IInd Symposium on Recent Advances in Plastic Surgery—RAPS 90,* March 28–30, 1990. Toledo LS, Pinto EBS (Eds.), Marques Saraiva, São Paulo, Brazil, 1990, p. 446.
9. Klein J: Tumescent technique. Am J Cosmetic Surg 4:263, 1987.
10. Toledo LS: Lipoescultura superficial. In: *Anestesia Locoregional em Cirurgia Estética.* Avelar JM (Ed.). Editora Hipócrates, São Paulo, Brazil 1993.
11. McKay W, Morris R, Mushlin P: Sodium bicarbonate attenuates pain on skin infiltration with lidocaine with or without epinephrine. Anesth Analg 66:572, 1987.
12. Gumucio CA, Bennie JB, Fernando B, Young VL, Roa N, Kraemer BA: Plasma lidocaine levels during augmentation mammaplasty and suction-assisted lipectomy. Plast Reconstr Surg 84(4):624, 1989.
13. Barnhart ER (Ed.): *Physician's Desk Reference.* Medical Economics Company, Inc., Oradell, New Jersey, 1989, p. 640.
14. Lillis PJ: Liposuction surgery under local anesthesia: Limited blood loss and minimal lidocaine absorption. J Dermatol Surg Oncol 14:10, 1988.
15. Teimourian B, Massac E Jr, Weigering CE: Reduction suction mammoplasty and suction lipectomy as an adjunct to breast surgery. Aesth Plast Surg 9:97, 1985.
16. Avelar JM, Illouz YG: In: *Lipoaspiração.* Editora Hipócrates, São Paulo, Brazil, 1986, pp. 148–152.
17. Mitnick JS, Roses DF, Harris MN, Colen SR: Calcifications of the breast after reduction mammoplasty. Surg Gynecol Obstet 17(5):409, 1990.
18. Buhtz C, Freitag J, Berge G, Pohl G: Mammographische Befunde nach Mammareduktionsplastik [Mammographic findings following reduction mammoplasty]. Zentralbl Chir 114(1):36, 1989.
19. Cruz NI, Guerrero A, Gonzalez CI: Current findings in the pathological evaluation of breast reduction specimens. Bol Assoc Med PR 81(10):387, 1989.
20. Clugston PA, Son-Hing QR, MacFarlane JK: Detecting breast cancer after reduction mammoplasty. Can J Surg 34(1):37, 1991.
21. Perras C: Fifteen years of mammography in cosmetic surgery of the breast. Aesth Plast Surg 14(2):81, 1990.
22. Cathcart RS III, Hagerty RC: Preoperative and postoperative considerations in elective breast operations. Ann Plast Surg 22(6):533, 1989.
23. Pinnella JW: Creating an inframammary crease with a liposuction cannula [letter]. Plast Reconstr Surg 83(5):925, 1989.
24. Vinnik CA: Suction lipoplasty of silicone-injected breasts: A warning [letter]. Plast Reconstr Surg 83(5):926, 1989.
25. Drever JM: Suction lipectomy: An excellent adjutant to improve the results of breast reconstruction with RAM flaps. Aesth Plast Surg 14(4):275, 1990.
26. Erol OO: Periareolar mammoplasty. In: *Annals of the IInd International Symposium on Recent Advances in Plastic Surgery—RAPS 92,* March 14–15, 1992. Toledo LS (Ed.), Estadão, São Paulo, Brazil, 1992, p. 103.
27. Matarasso A, Courtiss EH: Suction mammaplasty: The use of suction lipectomy to reduce large breasts. Plast Reconstr Surg 87(4):709, 1991.
28. Samdal F: The female breast and reduction liposculpture. In: *Liposculpture: The Syringe Technique.* Fournier P (Ed.). Arnette, Paris, 1991, p. 233.
29. Grazer FM: In: *Atlas of Suction Assisted Lipectomy.* Churchill Livingstone, New York, 1992, p. 141.
30. Illouz YG: In: *Body Sculpturing by Lipoplasty.* Churchill Livingstone, New York, 1989, p. 284.
31. Aiache A: Lipoplasty of the female breast. In: *Lipoplasty: The Theory and Practice of Blunt Suction Lipectomy.* Hetter GP (Ed.). Little, Brown, Boston, 1990, p. 305.
32. Stark GB, Grandel S, Spilker G: Tissue suction of the male and female breast. Aesth Plast Surg 16(4):317, 1992.

Role of Lollipop Excision

Introduction

Tolbert S. Wilkinson

Avoiding scars in the inframammary fold and interrupting neurovascular supply to a minimal degree have always been the goals of surgeons who address the problem of voluminous or ptotic breasts. Obviously if the breast can be restored to an acceptable position without skin removal, the results are aesthetically more pleasing and the complications are diminished. This is particularly important to those women who need a breast lift. They are more attuned to aesthetics than our reduction patients, and more critical of scarring. In the technique of breast infolding, the gland is reset at a higher position and the skin incision is limited to only that required to free the gland and infold it on itself.

For the American patient, this often leaves a breast that is too small, although well projecting. We choose to add a breast prosthesis for most of these cases. When an augmentation is added the breast tissue is overlapped left to right for added reinforcement, rather than infolded. Again, a short periareolar incision is the only requirement. In other cases, skin excision and areolar lifting are the better choice. The additional surgical maneuvers to minimize expansion of the areola and unacceptable periareolar scarring are even more important in the augmented mastopexy. Unless there is practically no subcutaneous tissue or breast tissue that can be used for the infolding or overlapping, the circumareolar mastopexy/augmentation is a better choice than a standard mastopexy.

Most mastopexy patients, unlike reduction patients, require a smaller circle that is to be deepithelialized. I have not had to employ the "lollipop" skin excision, a wedge excision of skin to give a tighter contour around the areola. Adding the lollipop vertical excision does decrease the complexity of the operation. However, I would prefer to limit this maneuver to the larger breast reductions in which skin tone is not ideal for the circle procedure.

All of the authors of this book have dealt with unpredictable scarring in the periareolar area. Unfortunately, in other breast surgeries with circumareolar incisions, we see the same scarring in the periareolar area as with standard inverted T surgeries. Revisions may be necessary, but with increasing familiarity and expertise in the performance of the circumareolar mastopexy, the scar revisions will be required less often.

Role of the Lollipop Conversion

Adrien Aiache

Unsatisfactory cases of circumareolar mastopexy include the following:

1. Breast mound truncated, flat, deformed, and not projected, leading to an unnatural appearance of the breast.
2. Poor circumareolar scarring with sunburst deformity of the areola with multiple, irregular areolar scars, stretching of the areola, paralysis of the areola-nipple complex leading to poor nipple projection, and irregular, inverted scars
3. Breast not well corrected with still unsatisfactory ptosis owing to a too-long infraareolar flap

The role of the lollipop conversion is to create a proper-appearing breast mound and areola with an acceptable, fine scar devoid of problems. The main complication encountered during lollipop conversion has been the difficulty in achieving skin approximation immediately below the areola; this is because a wide excision of skin has been performed and there is only a scant amount of skin left under the areola where the closure becomes tight (Figure 6.1).

Technique

It is necessary to include the circumareolar scar in the lollipop conversion in order to shift the tension to the skin area situated just below the areola, thus ensuring a fine areolar scar free of tension, and obtain good support below.

Unless only a small doughnut of skin has been excised, it will be difficult to obtain proper projection of the breast mound, owing to the paucity of skin in the immediate periareolar area (Figure 6.1A).

The circular scar is excised with two incisions within the areola and on the outer skin side. At the lower border, the skin is incised in the center and undermined for its approximation under the areola after proper excision has been done (Figure 6.1B). It could often be the tightest part of the areola because this is the greatest distance between the two skin borders and thus extensive undermining might be necessary for approximation.

In short, the lollipop conversion is performed essentially because of its scar improvement and secondary mound shape improvement, once the patient has understood and agreed to the inferior vertical scar obtained by this technique. If the breast is very large, it could even be necessary to transform the lollipop to an inverted T, because an excess of inframammary tissue might be present; excision of this tissue yields a horizontal submammary scar.

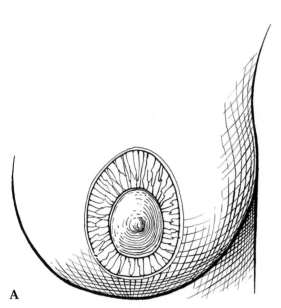

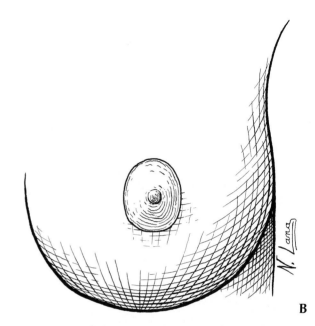

A

B

Figure 6.1. (A) The circumareolar (so-called doughnut) technique, in which a large circular segment of skin around the areola is excised. **(B)** The idealized scar obtained by this technique. **(C)** The lollipop conversion necessary when a larger amount of skin is excised and the circumareolar scar would not be acceptable. **(D)** Lollipop conversion allows tightening of the infraareolar skin, thus relaxing the actual circumareolar skin from tension and allowing a 1:1 length approximation of the sutures around the areola; the elevation and support of the breast and the scar are obtained by the vertical infraareolar scar. **(E)** If the breast is too large and the infraareolar area is extensive, an extension of the excision to the inframammary region will, in turn, give an inverted T scar. **(F)** The inverted T scar, or anchor scar, is shown after excising and suturing a large amount of skin and often breast tissue in the inframammary area.

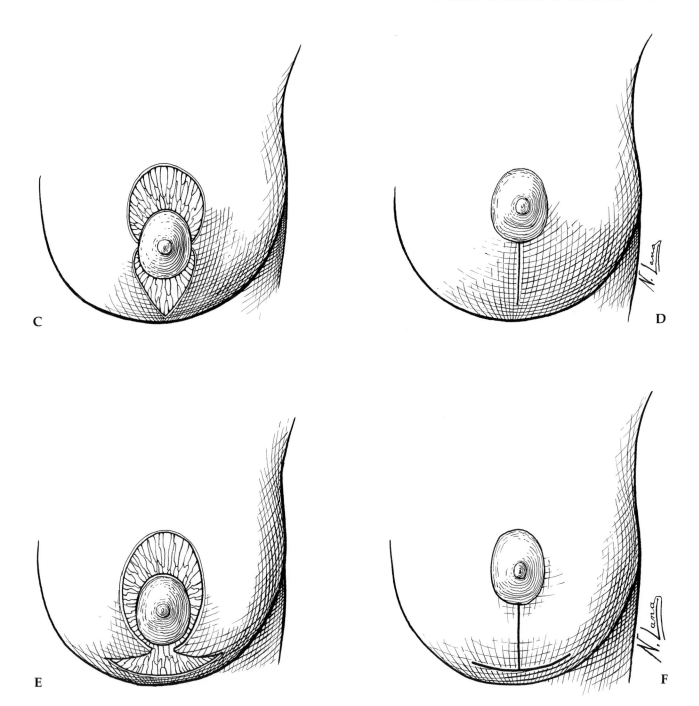

Mastopexy

Tolbert S. Wilkinson, Adrien Aiache, and Luiz S. Toledo

Introduction

Tolbert S. Wilkinson

Certain patients who require mastopexy are simply not candidates for the circumareolar technique, particularly if they have suffered attenuation of the breast skin and parenchyma. These women typically give a history of extreme swelling during pregnancy, which accentuates a pre-existing ptosis. The patient illustrated in Figure 7.1 is one such case. After pregnancy her breasts dropped to a lower position but without areolar expansion. A contracture is present on the right side. For this patient, the best technique is the "standard" but modified mastopexy in which the central portion of the inverted T is deepithelialized and used as reinforcement. Standard mastopexy markings are used, similar to those used for a McKissock breast reduction. The central zone and the area around the areola are deepithelialized so that they may offer further support. Entry is made from this point into the capsule and a new, wider based prosthesis of the textured type, is inserted. After the areola has been moved to its new elevated position, the lateral flaps are undermined and brought over the deepithelialized central portion. This double reinforcement gives the result shown in Figure 7.2. A short horizontal incision is used so that the excess skin may be gathered at the inverted T position at six o'clock, directly beneath the breast fold, thus minimizing problems with scar hypertrophy and widening.

Other patients may require repositioning of breast tissue but do not wish their breasts to be enlarged. One such case is shown in Figure 7.3. Notice the bizarre asymmetry of the breast and the inverted nipples. The patient is an actress and frequently wears revealing clothing. She was most insistent that the circumareolar technique be used but requested only elevation and reshaping. This technique is identical to those described in the South American literature and is less complicated than circumareolar reduction.

After manually infolding the breast in the preoperative consultation, the circle to be deepithelialized was drawn as shown in Figure 7.3A–C. A moderate reduction in areolar size was also dotted in, to be redrawn in the operating room. We also planned for this patient a simple epithelial excision within the separated nipple points, and simple closure with advancement of skin.

Operative photographs (Figures 7.4 through 7.10) show the progression of this procedure.

In Figure 7.4 the incisions are made to reduce

Figure 7.1. A candidate for a standard (noncircumareolar) mastopexy. The patient experienced extreme swelling during pregnancy, which exacerbated a preexisting ptosis. Attenuation of breast skin and parenchyma made her a less than ideal candidate for circumareolar mastopexy.

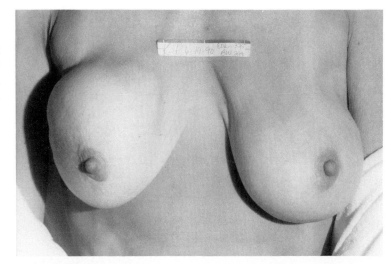

Figure 7.2. The same patient as in Figure 7.1, after the standard mastopexy had been performed.

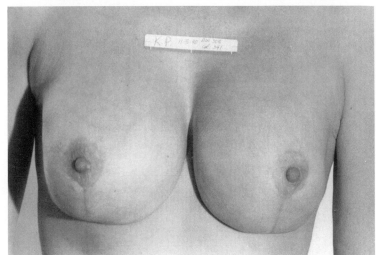

the relatively normal areolar diameter to 3.8 cm. The entire circle is deepithelialized.

In Figure 7.5 the breast tissue has been dissected away from the breast mound, using curved, blunt scissors for spreading and cutting. Note that fat is left on the undersurface for contouring and to assure a better blood supply. The nipple has now been moved into position with the triangle excision, and the breast mound is held in its new position with the curved retractor.

Figure 7.6 shows the first placement of the suture that anchors the breast mound in its new position. When the areola is centered, I have left a distance of 6 cm, which means the original length of areola to inframammary fold has been reduced.

Figure 7.7 shows the completion of the infolding sutures that have already been placed with the breast manually folded in and repositioned. A lattice of absorbable and nonabsorbable sutures creates the subcutaneous cone.

Figure 7.8 shows the breast mound completed with the nipple at its new position. Now a certain amount of additional dissection beneath the skin becomes necessary, so that the skin will drape to the new mound. Because of contracture and folding of the lower skin into the higher inframammary fold, we have left a 9-cm skin flap at this point. Figure 7.9 shows the appearance of the breast as the first circumareolar suture is placed. The final gaping shown at five o'clock will be gathered with the last two passes of the suture before it is tied, leaving an excess folding in the

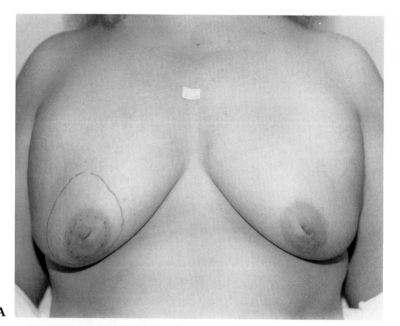

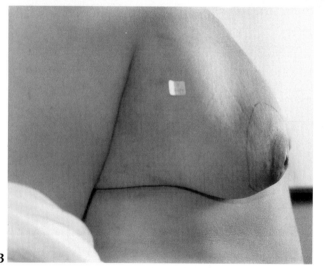

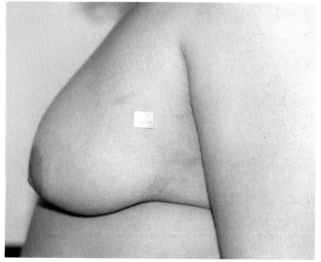

Figure 7.3. This patient requested only elevation and reshaping, without enlargement.

A

B

C

Figure 7.4. through 7.10 A series of operative photographs detailing the steps undertaken in the treatment of the patient shown in Figure 7.3. See text for details.

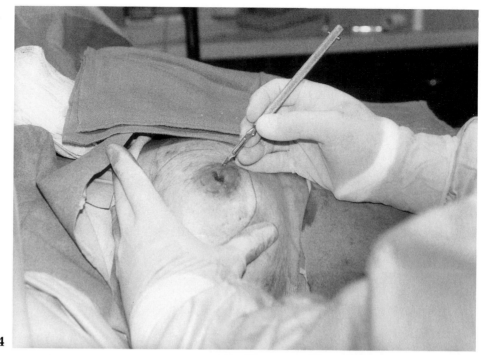

Figure 7.4

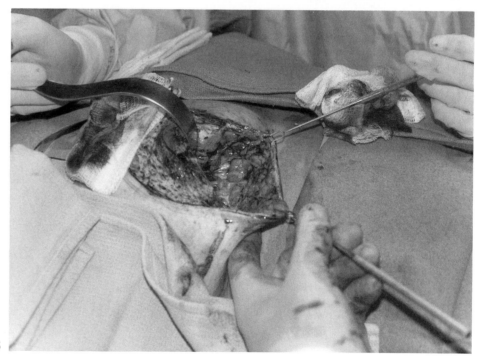

Figure 7.5

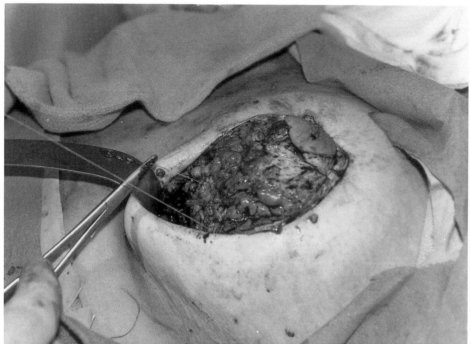

Figure 7.6

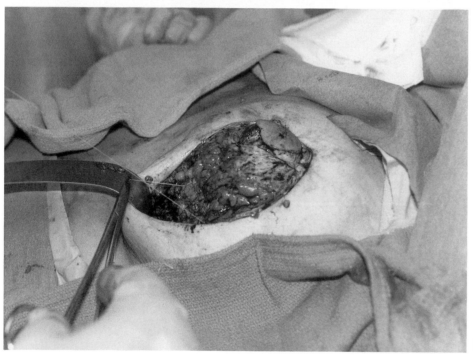

Figure 7.7

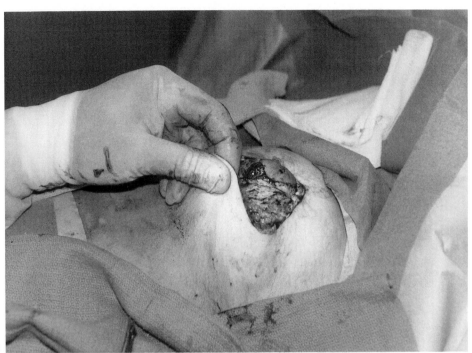

Figure 7.8

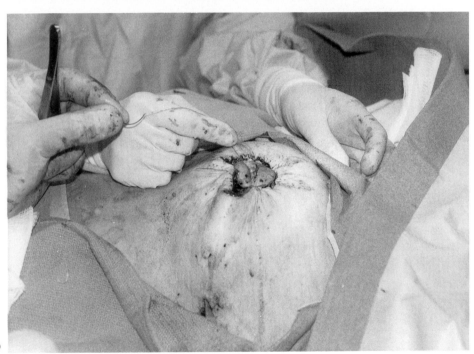

Figure 7.9

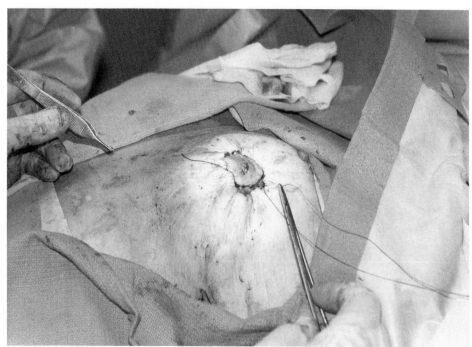

Figure 7.10

lower third of the breast. This favorable position receives the pressure of the breast weight against the brassiere and hastens resolution of the folding. The approximation of breast skin to areolar edge is completed with the second circumareolar suture of absorbable material. The original suture is tied below the surface and the end is left long. As we complete the circle, the end of the suture will be tied to the original knot at a distance of 0.5 cm below the everted skin edges (Figure 7.10). The placing of a circular PDS 2-0 suture around the base of the areola is another method of reducing late areolar stretch.

This, in a nutshell, is the technique used for mastopexy, reduction, and internal repair when there is an excess of skin and a greater degree of ptosis that requires nipple areolar repositioning.

Mammoplasty Using Syringe Liposuction and Periareolar Incision: An 8-Year Evolution

Luiz S. Toledo

Mastopexy

In the late 1980s important innovations improved the scope of reduction mammoplasty and mastopexy. The return of the periareolar incision and the introduction of liposuction,[1] and later syringe liposculpture,[2] are some of the technical advances that allowed us to provide shape improvement and shorter scars. Liposuction disproved the old concept that, to change form, a long incision is necessary. In the same way we were able to change the indication for abdomen dermolipectomies, we could also apply the same principles to breast surgery. Many breast hypertrophies are caused by excess fat. It is possible today to reduce fatty breasts considerably by liposuction alone, without the need for any other incisions.

In 1985 Brazilian mammoplasty patients became aware, by way of a glossy magazine article directed toward women, of a reduction mammoplasty technique with a single periareolar incision. In a country where the Pitanguy breast reduction technique, with its inverted T scar,[3] was employed by most surgeons, this news had great repercussions and patients started asking for the new procedure. My first potential periareolar patient presented me with the article and pressured me to try the procedure. I performed liposuction of the breast with the liposuction machine, resected gland tissue only in the lower part of the breast, and removed skin at the end of the procedure. We had agreed that if we did not like the shape obtained, we could always utilize the inverted T incision to correct the problem. This is one of the great advantages of the periareolar technique: you don't "burn your bridges," it can always be transformed into a vertical or an inverted T incision if required. The results were quite acceptable and this encouraged us to perfect the technique and present our findings at the ISAPS (International Society for Aesthetic Plastic Surgery) meeting in New York in 1987,[4,5] with a 1-year follow-up. By 1988[6] we were using the syringe in all our facial and body liposuction work. The syringe gave us more precision, and we started resecting gland in the upper pole as well, to elevate the areola in larger breasts. In 1989[7] we were resecting an oval of skin before gland resection and using the purse-string stitch around the areola to help prevent areolar enlargement.

Two major problems are associated with the periareolar incision: enlargement of the areola and recurrent breast ptosis. The inverted T scar was considered "the price" patients had to pay to obtain a well-shaped breast. Scars can become almost imperceptible with the years, but, depending on several factors, they will be more or less visible. We still use this procedure often, depending on the indication.

Method

We indicate the periareolar technique for breast reduction and mastopexy, mastopexy without reduction, and mastopexy with augmentation. Preoperative examinations should include a mammography. It has been reported that early diagnosis of breast cancer, during routine preoperative mammography, occurs in 2.9% of patients undergoing cosmetic surgery of the breast. These patients have a far better prognosis owing to the early detection of the disease.[8]

With a fatty breast, we begin the breast reduction or mastopexy procedure by reducing its size by syringe liposuction. Through an incision in the submammary fold we introduce a 20- to 35-cm-long, 3 to 5 mm-gauge "pyramid" tip cannula connected to a 60-cm^3 Toomey tip disposable syringe, filled with 5 cm^3 of Ringer's solution. The plunger is locked, creating a vacuum. Through this incision (Figure 7.11) the cannula

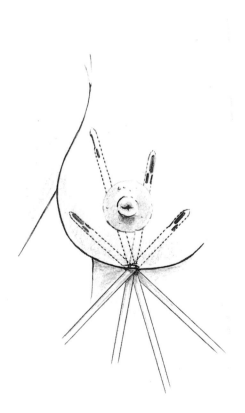

Figure 7.11. Cannula incision at the submammary fold.

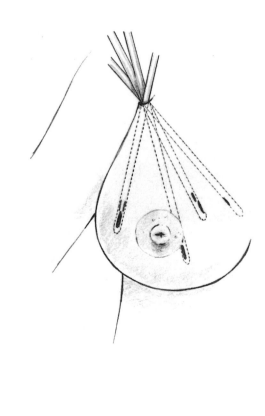

Figure 7.12. Cannula incision in the axilla, allowing for the criss-crossing of tunnels.

can reach the medial and lateral part of the breast, the axillary fold, and the base of the mammary cone. Another incision in the axilla (Figure 7.12) allows criss-crossing of the tunnels, for regularity.

Suction allows us to operate on a smaller breast, and therefore we always redo the markings because they will alter with the reduced size. Patients should be marked while seated. We first mark the new position and size of the areola and the amount of skin to be removed around it. We mark points A, B, and C, as in the Pitanguy technique (Figure 7.13). Point D is at a distance of approximately 5 to 6 cm from the submammary fold (Figure 7.14). Points are joined with an oval line, marking the excess skin to be removed; we are always careful not to resect too much skin, the cause of many of the problems related to this technique. The skin to be excised is deepithelialized, leaving a dermal pedicle around the areola (Figure 7.15). Through the oval incision we can

reach the mammary gland and dissect it from the skin, leaving a superior pedicle attached to the pectoral muscle. We dissect the inferior half of the gland away from the pectoral muscle (Figure 7.16), leaving it free to rotate and be elevated.

If after suction there is still a need for glandular removal, we calculate and resect a slice of gland from the inferior pole (Figure 7.17A). By suturing the edges with nonabsorbable stitches we obtain a smaller mammary cone, which will be sutured to the muscle and the rib periosteum in the correct position (Figure 7.17B). We can repeat this infolding procedure several times to obtain the breast firmness we desire.

If the areola is placed too low or is pointing downward after the resection and suture, we can lift the complex by resecting a pyramid, or prism, of gland from the upper pole. This should be done with extreme care in the area between the lateral and medial mammary branches, so as not to affect the pedicle of the breast (Figure 7.18A and B).

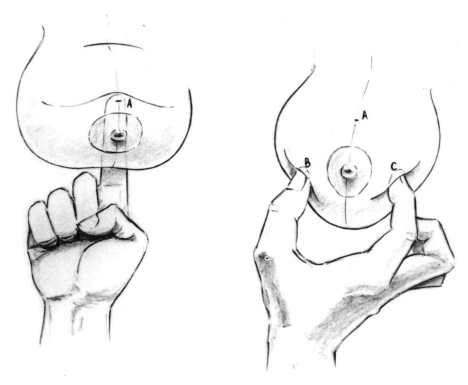

Figure 7.13. The marking of points A, B, and C, as in the Pitanguy technique.

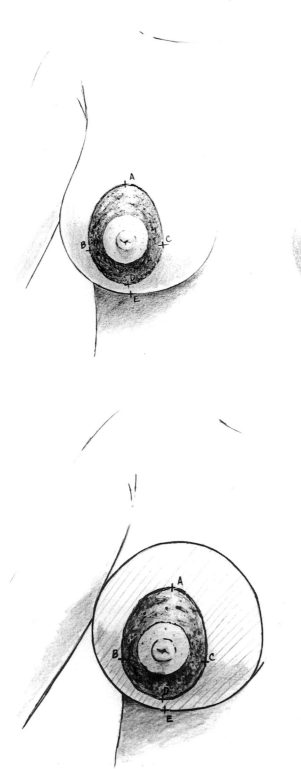

Figure 7.14. The marking of point D, at 5 to 6 cm from the mammary fold.

Figure 7.15. The oval of skin formed by the joining of points A, B, C, and D is deepithelialized, leaving a dermal pedicle around the areola. The remaining skin of the breast is dissected from the gland.

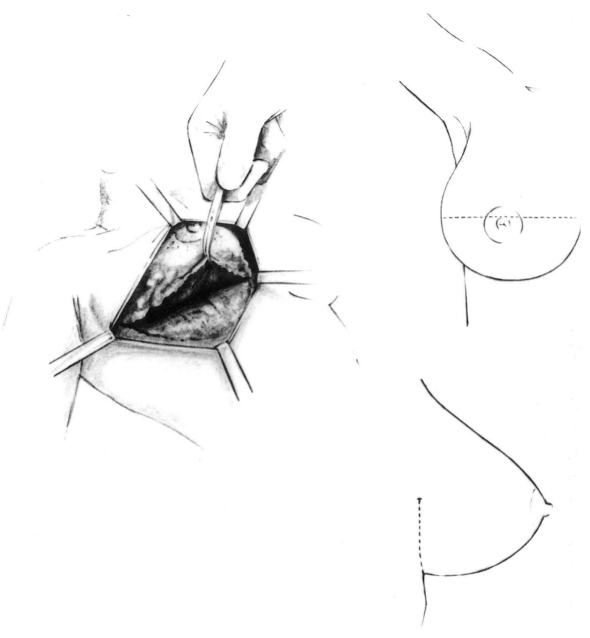

Figure 7.16. Dissection of the inferior half of the gland from the pectoral muscle.

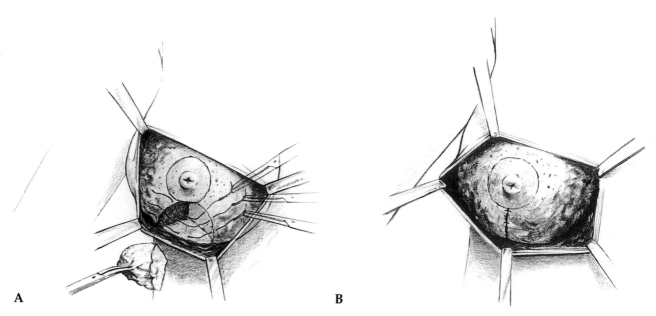

Figure 7.17. **(A)** Resection of a slice of gland from the inferior pole. **(B)** The two flaps are rotated and sutured in the midline and secured to the pectoral muscle and rib periosteum.

The dermal flap is sutured with a purse-string multifilament stitch (Mersilene 0) around the areola, allowing for a better shape and size of the areola (Figure 7.19). Skin is sutured to the areola with separate Nylon 5-0 stitches. Suction drains are placed because of the skin dissection.

If there is no need for fat reduction we start the procedure with the periareolar incision. For mastopexy alone, gland is not removed and through the same incision we reposition the breast. For mastopexy with augmentation we perform the mastopexy in the usual manner and insert a silicone prosthesis (Figure 7.20) to augment the breast, and to improve the shape and projection (Figure 7.21A and B). Women in Brazil and Europe prefer smaller breasts. We rarely use a prosthesis larger than 200 cm^3, usually between 100 and 160 cm^3 per breast.

Figure 7.18. (A) Resection of a pyramid, or prism, of gland from the upper pole. **(B)** Suture of the upper pole, elevating the nipple-areolar complex.

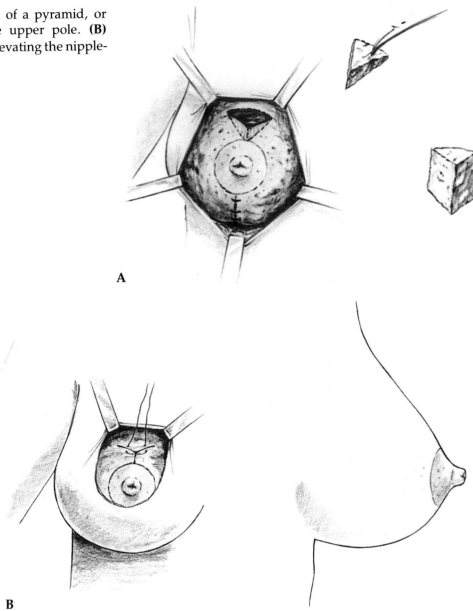

A

B

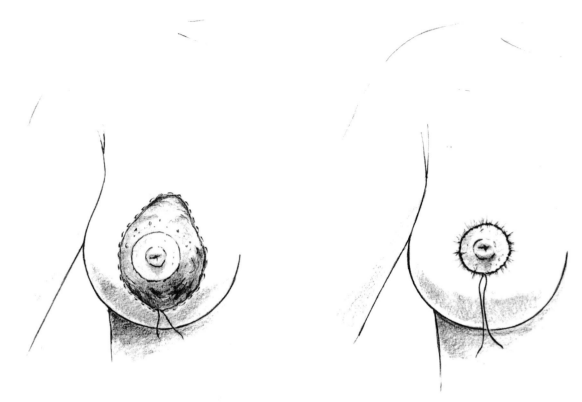

Figure 7.19. The purse-string multifilament stitch reduces the outer circle to the areola diameter.

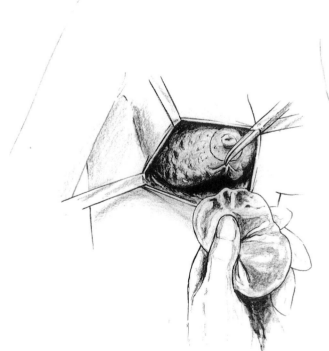

Figure 7.20. Mastopexy with augmentation, using a silicone prosthesis.

Figure 7.21. **(A)** Preoperative appearance of a 25-year-old patient with breast ptosis and areolar enlargement. **(B)** Four months postoperatively, after mastopexy, augmentation, and areolar reduction.

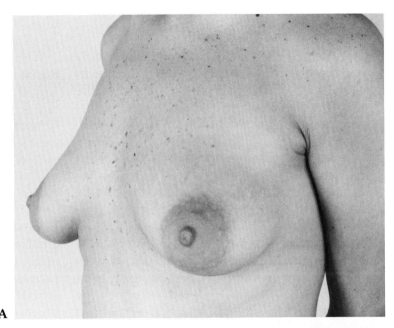

A

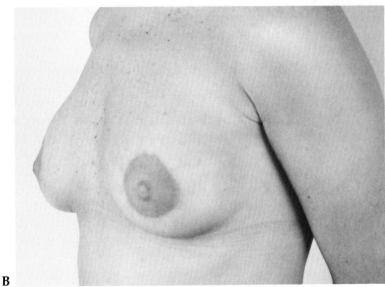

B

Discussion

We indicate the periareolar technique in very specific cases. A candidate for breast reduction or mastopexy is shown two examples of breasts: the first is pear shaped, with a very projected nipple-areolar complex; the second is rounder in shape, with a flattened areola. The patient is asked which type of breast she prefers. If the patient prefers a round breast we indicate the periareolar technique, because this is the type of result we will obtain. We indicate the periareolar technique for (1) patients who will not benefit from suction alone, (2) patients who prefer the more rounded breast example, (3) young patients who plan to breast feed or who are still subject to a change of breast shape, (4) young patients with posture problems, and (5) patients who will not accept the inverted T incision. All these patients are made aware that they might need to undergo a second procedure in the future.

If we use the inverted T incision, we try to keep the horizontal scar as short as possible and within the inframammary crease area. Excessive concern over the final scar should not interfere with the final results of the mammoplasty, as far as shape, volume, and lasting results are concerned.[9]

We advocate the inverted T technique for (1) patients who prefer a pear-shaped breast, even if they are young. These patients will never be happy with the periareolar result, because the technique will not produce this breast shape; (2) patients with posture problems and back pain, who are not concerned with the size of the scar; (3) older patients who no longer wear bathing suits; (4) out-of-town patients, who want a fast recovery time.

With an inverted T reduction we remove the stitches around the seventh postoperative day, and the usual follow-up procedure is quite simple. The periareolar technique patients, on the other hand, require a longer, more complicated postoperative follow-up. It is usual for these patients to have to return many times over several weeks for dressing changes, depending on the amount of periareolar wrinkling. Some patients return to the office weekly for a period of 6 months. We avoid the periareolar technique in cases of severe ptosis or hypertrophy.

With time and consecutive pregnancies, the breast tends to become bigger and heavier, more flaccid and ptotic. Breast ptosis after breast reduction is twice as frequent among women who have been through pregnancy.[10] The main difference for these patients is that more skin needs to be removed, the areolar pedicle becomes too long, and there can be some difficulty in repositioning it. Special care is always taken to ensure possible future breast feeding. Depending on the degree of ptosis it might be difficult to reposition the areola while still maintaining the integrity of the milk ducts. The aesthetics and sensitivity of the breasts are very important to women and these functions should be preserved during aesthetic surgery. The sensitivity and feeding function of the nipple-areolar complex must be preserved. We have all of this in mind when we opt for a breast reduction technique.

In 1987,[4] when we first presented the technique with a 1-year follow-up, we were treating only mastopexy and small and medium hypertrophies (Figures 7.22 through 7.24). Skin was resected only when the breast was in its final shape and position. We found that resecting the skin at the end of the surgery provoked areolar asymmetries, which then had to be corrected (Figure 7.25). We stopped resecting skin completely by 1988,[6] and skin excess would usually accommodate to the new shape of the breast (Figure 7.26). In 1989 we realized that, by not removing skin, we were seeing early ptosis in patients in which the weight of the breast was too heavy to be supported by poor-quality skin. We began resecting skin at the beginning of surgery,[7] before the gland resection, and we used the purse-string stitch around the areola (Figure 7.27).

We soon realized that gland resection of the lower pole (caudal) did not correct the whole breast and in some cases the breast was left "looking downward," even with fat suction. We started removing a prism- or pyramid-shaped piece of gland from the upper pole, suturing in such a way as to elevate the areola (Figure 7.28). This resection has the same effect as the keel of the Pitanguy technique,[3] and allowed us to treat

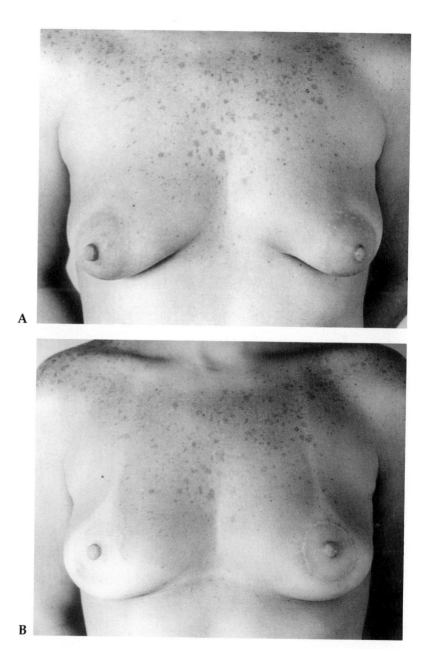

Figure 7.22. (A) Preoperative appearance of a 36-year-old patient with breast ptosis and small hypertrophy. (B) The same patient postoperatively, after a small reduction and periareolar mastopexy.

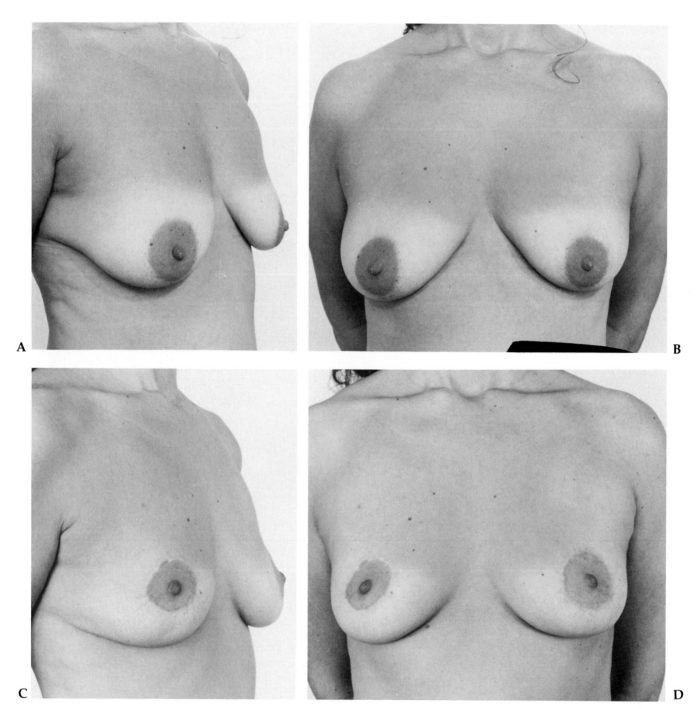

Figure 7.23. (A, B) Preoperative of a 32-year-old patient with breast ptosis and medium hypertrophy. **(C, D)** The same patient postoperatively, after periareolar mastopexy and breast reduction.

Figure 7.24 **(A)** Preoperative appearance of a 36-year-old patient with breast ptosis and medium hypertrophy. **(B)** One year postoperatively, after periareolar mastopexy and breast reduction. **(C)** Same patient 6 years postoperatively, after periareolar mastopexy and breast reduction.

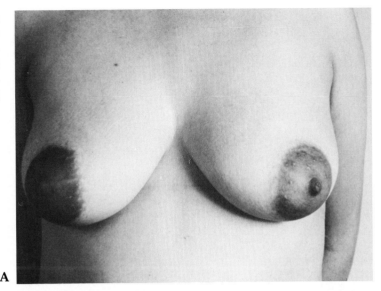

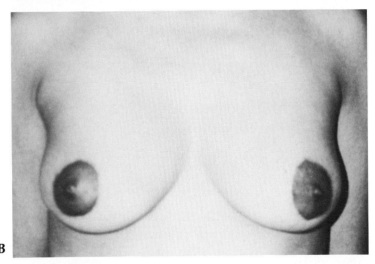

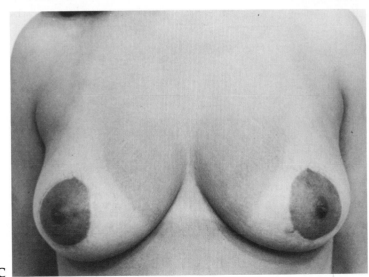

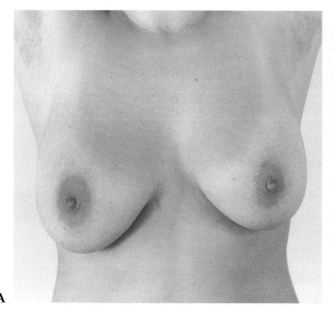

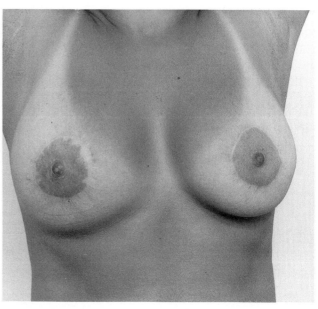

A B

Figure 7.25. (A) Preoperative appearance of a 37-year-old patient with breast ptosis and medium hypertrophy. **(B)** Six months postoperatively, after periareolar mastopexy and breast reduction. The patient developed areolar asymmetry and discoloration of the right areolar scar.

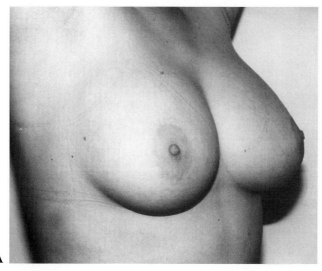

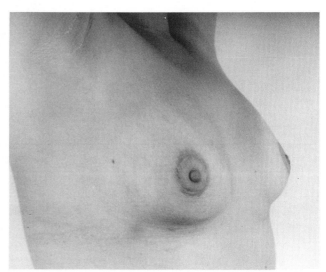

A B

Figure 7.26. (A) Preoperative appearance of an 18-year-old patient with fat and gland breast hypertrophy. **(B)** Six years postoperatively, after suction of 350 cm^3 of fat and 150 g of gland per breast. No skin was removed. The patient underwent two pregnancies and breast fed the two children during this period of time.

Figure 7.27. **(A)** Preoperative appearance of a 70-year-old patient with fat and gland breast hypertrophy and very flaccid skin. **(B)** One month postoperatively, after periareolar breast reduction and mastopexy. Skin excess was calculated and removed at the beginning of the procedure. A purse-string stitch was used around the areola.

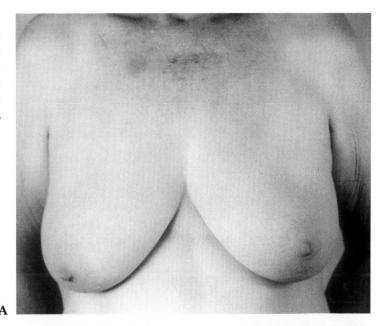

A

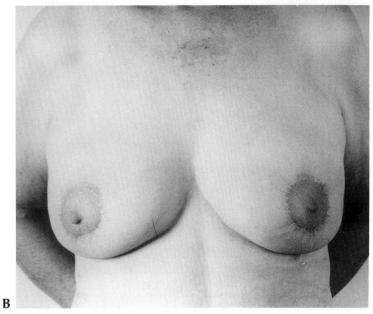

B

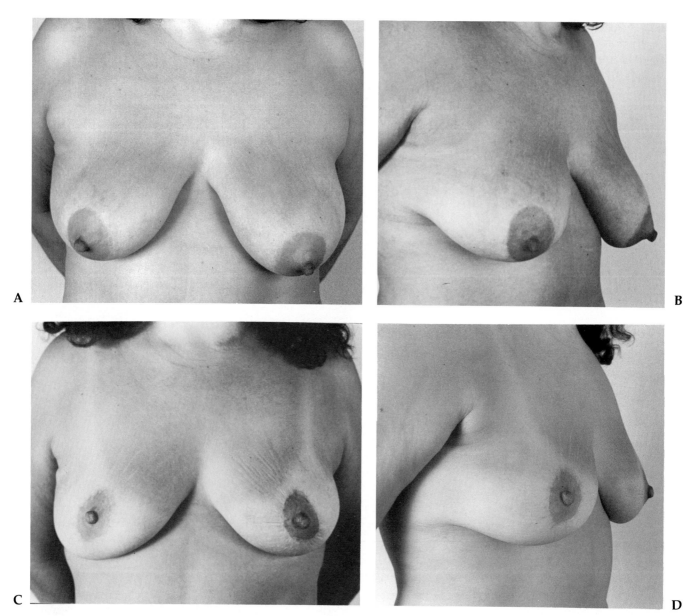

Figure 7.28. (A, B) Preoperative appearance of a 40-year-old patient with asymmetric breasts, fat and gland breast hypertrophy, and very flaccid skin and stretch marks. **(C, D)** The same patient postoperatively, after periareolar breast reduction and mastopexy. Skin excess was calculated and removed at the beginning of the procedure. A slice of gland was removed in the inferior pole, as well as a pyramid at the upper pole, to elevate the niplle-areolar complex. A purse-string stitch was used around each areola.

larger breasts. This prism of gland is removed only if needed, and only after the breast is sutured in place. We have been able to reshape large breasts successfully, removing up to 1 kg of fat and glandular tissue per breast (Figure 7.29), by first suctioning fat and then resecting gland through the incision.

The purse-string stitch gives us good roundness of the areola, but if we miscalculate the amount of skin to be resected we can end up with an oval areola. The outer concentric periareolar circle must be drawn not to exceed twice that of the inner areolar circle, to allow for the excision of a maximum amount of areola and periareolar

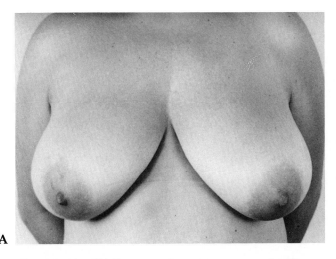 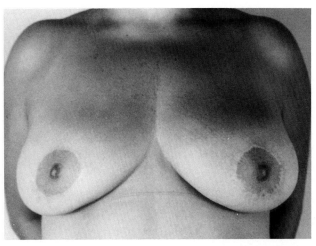

A   B

Figure 7.29. (A) Preoperative appearance of a 40-year-old patient with severe breast hypertrophy and ptosis. **(B)** The same patient postoperatively, after suction of 500 cm^3 of fat and removal of 500 g of gland per breast.

skin without the side effect of poor scars and enlarged areolae.[11] Limitations seem to be more evident in cases in which it is necessary to deepithelialize circles 11 to 12 cm in diameter.[12] Although skin pleating usually disappears in 2 to 4 months, it can sometimes take more than 6 months, in addition to our having to do scar revisions (Figure 7.30). This means a difficult postoperative period for both patient and doctor.

After performing the periareolar technique, the surgeon should follow the patient closely. Suction drains are removed around the third day, or when suction is less than 50 cm^3/24-hr period. After the removal of the drains, the wound is covered with Micropore tape (3M Company, Minneapolis, MN) and a shower is permitted. An elastic brassiere (with no seams) should be worn for 30 days. Patients should be warned against too much arm movement during the first 2 weeks; driving is not permitted. Stitches are removed between 7 and 10 days postoperatively.

There is usually no postoperative pain, only some tenderness in the first 24 hr, easily treated with analgesics. Swelling should decrease by 80% by the end of the first month, the remaining 20% by the sixth month. Bruising, when it occurs, lasts from 2 to 3 weeks. Manual lymphatic drainage is prescribed every other day for the first 10 days. This helps to accelerate the recovery time, reduce fluid retention, and eliminate discomfort.

Conclusion

The periareolar technique has one main advantage—only one incision is made, around the areola—and many disadvantages and pitfalls, which should be avoided at all costs to obtain a successful result. There is no benefit in using this single-incision technique if the final shape of the breast is unacceptable. We should not jeopardize the shape of the breast by indicating an inadequate technique because its scars are shorter. The major dilemma of reduction mammoplasty and mastopexy is the shape of the breast versus the size of the scar. With our technique, selected breasts can be reduced by liposuction, gland can be resected, and the mastopexy performed through a periareolar incision, resulting in virtually imperceptible scarring. Problems appeared only when we pushed the boundaries of the indications and attempted to treat breasts that were too big, too flaccid, or both. The results were lack of projection in the shape of the breast, and widening of the areola. Two examples for which an inverted T technique is indicated are presented in Figures 7.31 and 7.32.

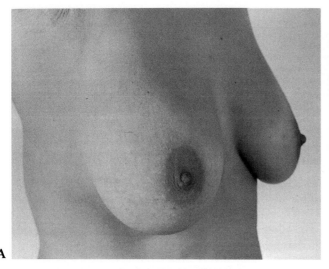
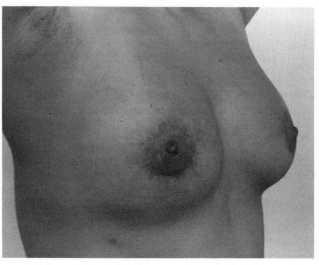

A
B

Figure 7.30. (A) Preoperative appearance of a candidate for periareolar mastopexy and reduction for medium hypertrophy. **(B)** The same patient postoperatively; pleating is apparent around the areola. To eliminate pleating we apply Micropore dressings daily for at least 2 months, if there are no signs of skin allergy.

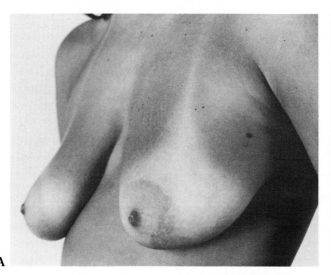
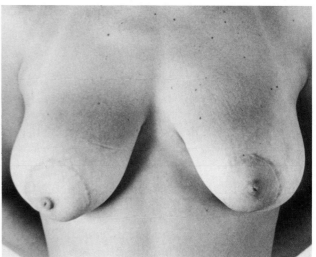

A
B

Figure 7.31. (A) An 18-year-old patient with medium hypertrophy, flaccid skin, and breast ptosis. Patient submitted to a periareolar mastopexy and 2 weeks later left to live in another country. **(B)** The same patient, 2 years postoperatively. She had undergone three pregnancies and miscarriages in that period of time. There was a complete return of the problem, plus a periareolar scar. **(C, D)** Same patient prior to an inverted T reduction and mastopexy. We opted for this technique because of her flaccidity and because we could not follow her for long postoperatively, as she could stay in the country for only 2 weeks. **(E)** Two weeks following an inverted T reduction mastopexy, using a short horizontal scar. **(F)** Two years postoperatively. Even with skin flaccidity, the result holds well and the shape of the breast is much better.

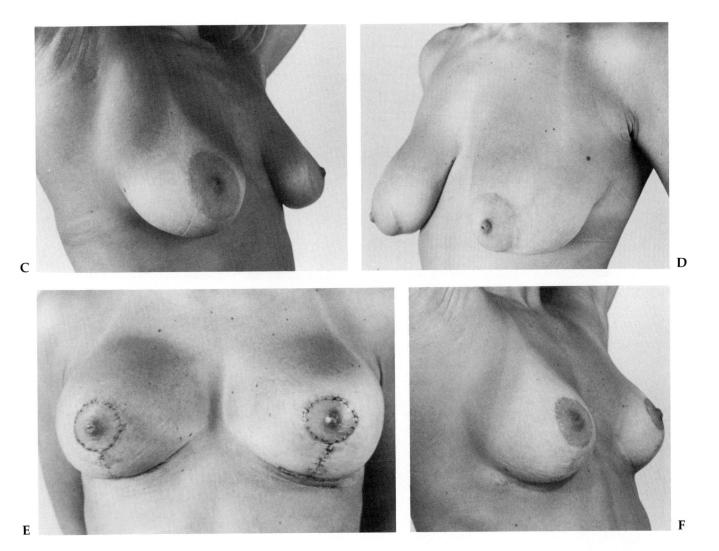

C

D

E

F

Figure 7.32

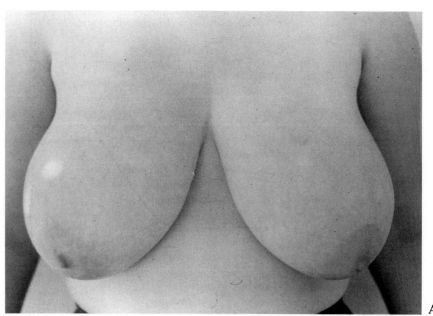

A

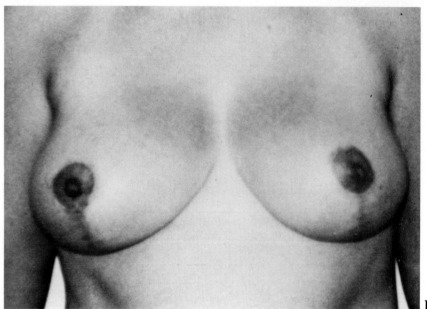

B

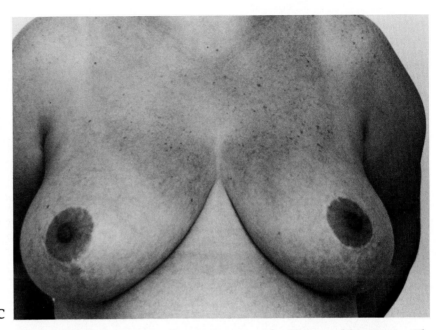

C

Figure 7.32. **(A)** Preoperative appearance of a 30-year-old patient with severe breast hypertrophy and ptosis. **(B)** One year after breast reduction and mastopexy, using an inverted T technique with short horizontal scar. **(C)** Eighteen years postoperatively. This patient had three pregnancies and breast fed three children in this period of time and put on 20 kg (40 lb). The result is still acceptable.

Comments

Adrien Aiache

It is certain that in mastopexy the problems associated with the doughnut-type excision and scarring will be relatively minimal because the breast tissue is not excessive and the weight of the tissue will not be an additional factor in scar formation, as it is when standard techniques are used. Cases suitable for mastopexy must be chosen carefully, because some relative deformity such as flattening of the breast mound and, possibly, nipple-areolar distortion may occur. However, it is in this sort of case that this technique is most satisfactory.

References

1. Illouz YG: Une nouvelle technique por les lipodistrophies localizes. Rev Chir Est Lang Franç 6:19, 1980.
2. Fournier P: *Liposculpture—Ma Technique.* Arnette, Paris, 1989.
3. Pitanguy I: Mamaplastias. Estudo de 234 casos consecutivos e apresentação de técnica pessoal. Rev Bras Cir Oct 1961.
4. Toledo LS, Matsudo PKR: Mammoplasty using liposuction and the periareolar incision. In: *Abstract Book of the IXth Congress of ISAPS.* New York, October 11–14, 1987, p. 35.
5. Toledo LS, Matsudo PKR: Mammoplasty using liposuction and periareolar incision. Aesth Plast Surg 13(1):9, 1989.
6. Toledo LS: Periareolar mammoplasty with syringe liposuction. In: *Annals of the International Symposium on Recent Advances in Plastic Surgery—RAPS 89,* March 3–5, 1989. Toledo LS (Ed.), Estadão, São Paulo, Brazil, 1989, p. 256.
7. Toledo LS: Mammoplasty using syringe liposuction and periareolar incision—a four year experience. In: Annals of the IInd International Symposium on Recent Advances in Plastic Surgery—RAPS 90. Revinter, São Paulo, Brazil, March 28–30, 1990, p. 127.
8. Perras C: Fifteen years of mammography in cosmetic surgery of the breast. Aesth Plast Surg 14(2):81, 1990.
9. de Pina DP: Mammaplasty: Shape, volume, and scar size. Aesth Plast Surg 14(1):27, 1990.
10. Aboudib JH Jr, de Castro CC, Coelho RS, Cupello AM: Analysis of late results in postpregnancy mammoplasty. Ann Plast Surg 26(2):111, 1991.
11. Spear SL, Kassan M, Little JW: Guidelines in concentric mastopexy. Plast Reconstr Surg 85(6):961, 1990.
12. Fogli A: Indications et limites du lifting du sein par voie peri-areolaire (round block). A propos de quarante-huit cas [Indications and limitations of breast lifting by periareolar approach (round block). Report of 48 cases]. Ann Chir Plast Esthet 35(6):459, 1990.

Circumareolar Mastopexy and Moderate Reduction

Adrien Aiache

In mastopexy the problems created by the dough-nut-type excision and scarring are relatively minimal, because the breast tissue is not excised and the weight of the tissue will not be an additional contributing factor in the final scar obtained by the circumareolar technique. Patients for whom mastopexy is indicated are chosen carefully because some deformity can be secondary to the technique. These deformities consist of flattening of the breast mound and nipple-areolar distortion, as well as inversion of the suture area and a protruding type of areola.

Reduction of Moderately Enlarged Breasts

Moderately enlarged breasts represent an important category of breast deformity that can be approached by varied surgical methods. What is considered a very moderate breast hypertrophy in this country is viewed as a large hypertrophy in Europe and South America, and the surgeon must recognize this to ensure that the patient understands the operation and the description of the size of the breast.

It is often mentioned by American plastic surgeons that what is considered a breast reduction overseas is viewed in this country as a simple mastopexy. Techniques such as those of Arie, Pitanguy, Marchac, Peixoto, and so on, are essentially devised for a mastopexy and could not be satisfactorily used in very large breast hypertrophies.

For moderate hypertrophy I have used a method based on the superior breast pedicle, as described in various journals. Smaller breasts are treated by crescent mastopexy and, if slightly larger, by a circumareolar mastopexy. If a patient rejects the telltale scars of mastopexy, the circumareolar technique can be used provided she understands the limitations of the technique and that the resulting shape could be less than ideal, as well as that the resulting circumareolar scar could be less than perfect.

Many techniques have been developed for the reduction of the moderately large breast. The scars obtained vary from the inverted T to the horizontal type of scar with circumareolar scarring.

Most of the accepted techniques at the time of this writing involve an operation based on the

119

upper or lower breast pedicle; some use a lateral pedicle. The resulting scars in moderately large breasts are often objectionable because the patients frequently desire a mastopexy correction, are not anxious to reduce the size of their breasts, and are not ready to accept excessive scarring in view of the mild nature of their problem. In these particular cases, the circumareolar mammoplasty can be adjusted with some mild reduction of the breast mound to give a more acceptable breast size and an acceptable scar. It is still possible to obtain results that would be acceptable in view of the fact that it would limit the extent of scarring. It is, however, in these cases that one should be more attentive to details to avoid potential problems secondary to this particular technique of circumareolar mastopexy.

Technique

The major steps of the circumareolar technique are outlined in Table 8.1, and described in greater detail below.

The nipple location is elected and the measurements made in relation to the amount of breast tissue present (Figure 8.1). If the breasts are large, it might be necessary to keep a distance of 6 to 7 cm below the areola and 12 to 13 cm on each side when measured from the areola to the midsternal line and midaxillary line. Proper inferior undermining of the lower and upper mounds allows the reduction in size in the center. More breast tissue can be removed to obtain the results desired.

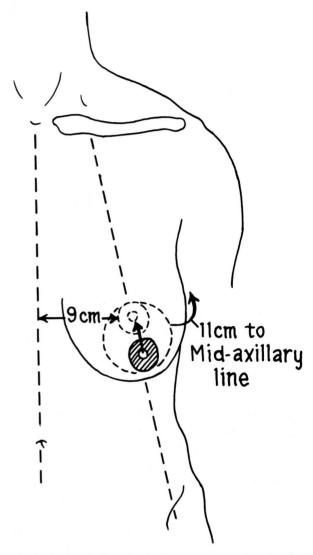

Figure 8.1. The circumareolar circle is drawn. The remaining width of skin after excision should not exceed 9 cm in length from the skin edge to the midsternal line and should not exceed 11 cm from the excised skin to the midaxillary line. Inferiorly, the inferior flap should not exceed 5 cm in distance from the inframammary line to the skin edge resection.

Table 8.1. Circumareolar mastopexy: Step by step

Step	Procedure
1.	Create markings
2.	Perform doughnut excision
3.	Undermine skin in all directions
4.	Reshape the breast mound:
	a. Excise central tissue, sometimes inferior horizontal tissue
	b. Reapproximate
	c. Excise superior keel of tissue
	d. Reapproximate superiorly the breast mound
5.	Perform circumareolar suturing
6.	Close the circle to the areola

The placement of the areola is determined by the superior limit of the circle to be excised from the breast. First, the nipple location is determined; it will depend on the size of the patient, the size of the chest wall (some patients have a long trunk and short legs), and the width of her shoulders. If the shoulders are broad, it is preferable to lower the nipple for proper appearance of the breast. In the lateral direction, the nipple is positioned on an oblique line extending from the middle third of the clavicle to the iliac crest. Notwithstanding the proper measurements (between 18 and 25 cm below the clavicle), the nipple location will often depend on the surgeon's taste and the patient's desire (Figure 8.2).

Once the nipple location is settled, a proper delineation of the areola is then decided; again, it will often depend on personal taste, tempered with some knowledge about the ideal size and proper size. Four to 4.5 cm seems to be a diameter agreed upon by most.

When the size of the areola has been determined, it is marked on the actual areola. If the breasts are full and tense, very little holding of the skin is necessary; however, if the breast are flat and empty, the areolar skin will shrink and the actual breast must be held under tension in order to allow the proper markings of the dimensions of the areolar circle. One must keep in mind that too much tension on the areola will stretch the muscle and prevent its proper contraction, especially when the periareolar permanent suture is inserted.

On the other hand, if the areola is strangled to a smaller circle by the periareolar suture, the orbicularis muscle will then bulge in a "Snoopy"-type deformity secondary to its concentric contracture. The overstretched muscle may end up partially paralyzed and unable to contract and allow protrusion of the nipple. Once the areolar dimension has been elected and the area of skin excision is marked, the main considerations are the following:

1. The outer and inner circle skin excisions are marked, keeping in mind the remaining skin that is necessary to obtain a properly shaped breast mound (4 to 9 cm medially, and 11 to 13 cm laterally, are the usual dimensions; it is prudent to keep in mind that whereas greater dimensions will not have any untoward effect, reduced dimensions of the medial and lateral walls will produce a flattened breast, which will then look truncated). The measurements are made from the midsternal line and from the midvertical axillary line. These measure-

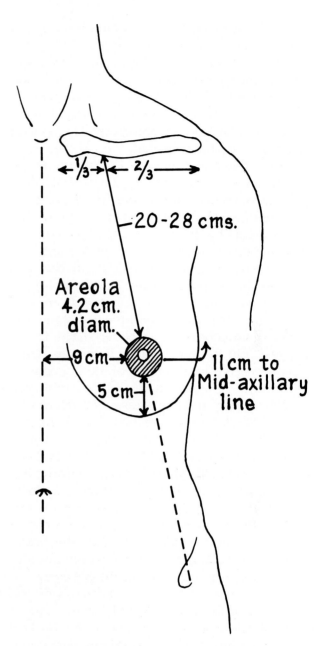

Figure 8.2. The accepted measurements for proper shape and location of the nipple-areolar complex and the breast mound. The areola varies in diameter from 3 to 5 cm, according to the size of the breast itself, the desires of the patient, and the surgeon's judgment. The nipple-areolar complex is located 20 to 28 cm below the clavicle mid-third point on the mammary line, going toward the iliac crest inferiorly. The areola is situated 9 cm from the midsternal line, 11 cm from the midaxillary line, and 5 cm from the inframammary line.

ments are important and should be properly made before the excisional surgery.

In addition to to contributing inordinately to the truncated appearance, a shortened skin cover will be difficult to modify and an eventual transformation of the circumareolar technique to a "lollipop" technique will be difficult if there is a paucity of skin.

2. Superiorly, it is preferable to undermine the skin to be able to allow a good repartition of the subcuticular suture and to ensure even distribution of the pleats created around the new areola by this technique, which consists of adapting a large circle to a smaller one.

3. Inferiorly, the limit of excision of the skin should be designed to leave an inferior lip of 5 to 6 cm of skin. These measurements are well accepted, because a short lip will distend and will eventually confer a better shape to the breast. On the other hand, if this lip is not properly reduced, ptosis of the mammary gland will certainly occur, and the nipple will ride too high. In large breasts, the inferior lip could be slightly longer than 5 to 6 cm, but usually it is better to leave this measurement smaller than expected. Once the skin has been excised medially, laterally, and inferiorly, it is necessary to undermine it, leaving a thick, fatty layer for proper vascularization. At this stage, the breast mound can be sculptured.

4. Exposure of the inferior part of the breast mound is obtained by proper skin undermining, similar in technique to the development of a flap in a subcutaneous mastectomy. Retraction of the flaps inferiorly allows proper visualization of the breast mound. A large keel of breast tissue is excised (Figure 8.3), often associated with a horizontal keel (thus perpendicular to the first one), leaving two lateral pillars of breast tissue (Figures 8.4 and 8.5). The volume of excision is determined by the need for reduction in each particular breast. The lateral pillars are then sutured in the middle, closing any potential dead space.

5. The skin flap is then developed superiorly, enough to assure a superior visualization of a keel excision with sufficient draping at the time of closure. Retraction of the skin flap superiorly allows the keel excision, which is

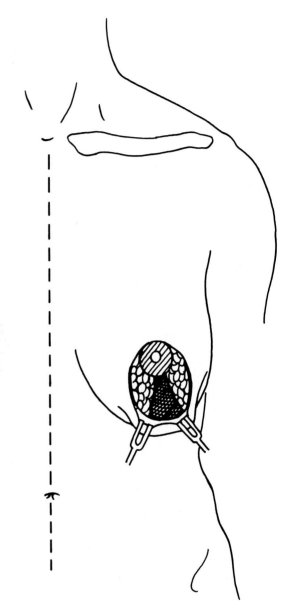

Figure 8.3. A segment of breast tissue is excised inferiorly for volume reduction. The breast tissue is excised in a vertical shape down to the pectoralis major.

necessary sometimes to obtain a reduction in breast size and a proper areolar relocation to a higher level (Figure 8.6). Once the defect has been closed, draping of the tissue is obtained, releasing any skin to gland attachments by extending the undermining as necessary.

6. Closure is accomplished as described in Chapter 4. Either absorbable sutures or permanent sutures are used for breast mound reconstruc-

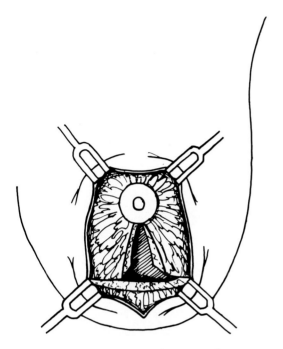

Figure 8.4. If necessary, a horizontal segment of breast tissue can be excised for further reduction in the size of the breast mound.

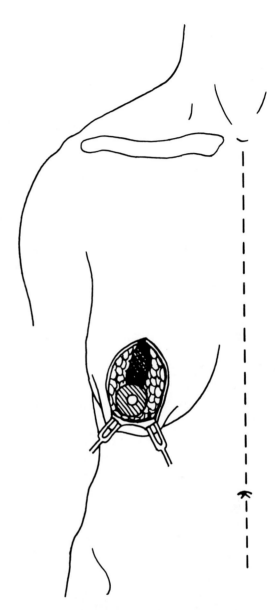

Figure 8.6. A superior keel of breast tissue can be excised as well, for elevation of the nipple, and for reduction in the size of the superior breast pole.

tion. The skin envelope is then draped over the reconstructed mound and the purse-string suture is applied and tightened to the dimensions desired. A metallic circle of the proper dimension can be used for exact measurement of the circle and exact tightening around the circle. The permanent suture is then followed by a row of subcuticular sutures and a third row for skin closure. Figures 8.7 through 8.14 show cases of mastopexy, breast reduction, and augmentation.

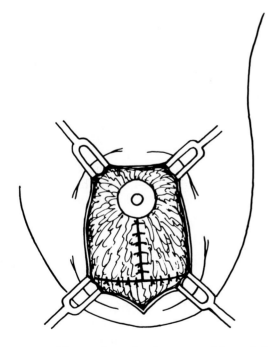

Figure 8.5. Shown here is the type of breast tissue reconstruction obtained by the inferior mammary excision associated with the vertical breast excision, thus reducing the size of the breast mound.

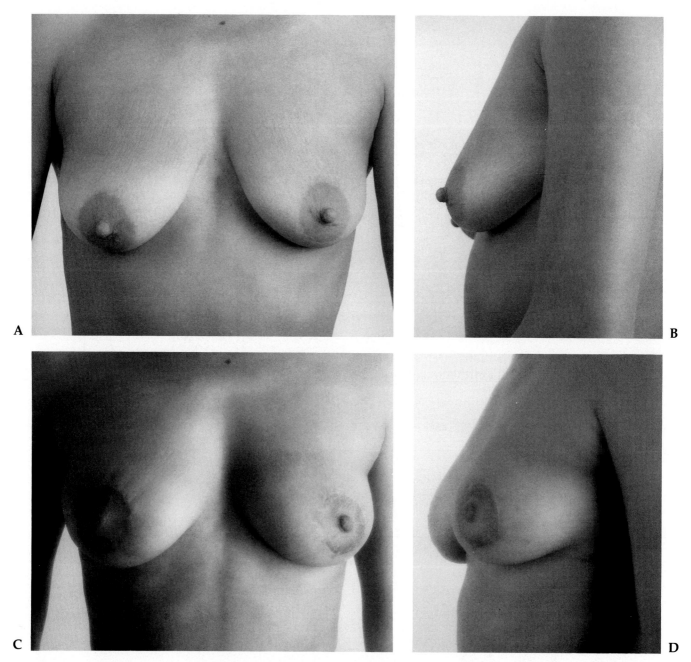

Figure 8.7. **(A)** Frontal and **(B)** lateral preoperative views of a 27-year-old woman with breast ptosis. **(C, D)** Postoperative appearance after circumareolar mammoplasty: **(C)** frontal; **(D)** lateral.

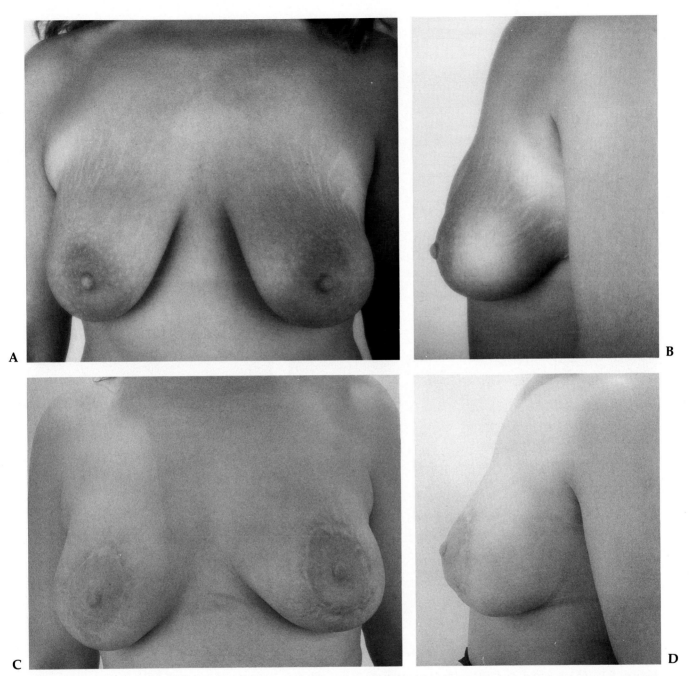

Figure 8.8. **(A)** Frontal and **(B)** lateral preoperative views of a 28-year-old woman with breast ptosis and hypotrophy. **(C, D)** Postoperative appearance after breast implantation and circumareolar mammoplasty: **(C)** frontal; **(D)** lateral.

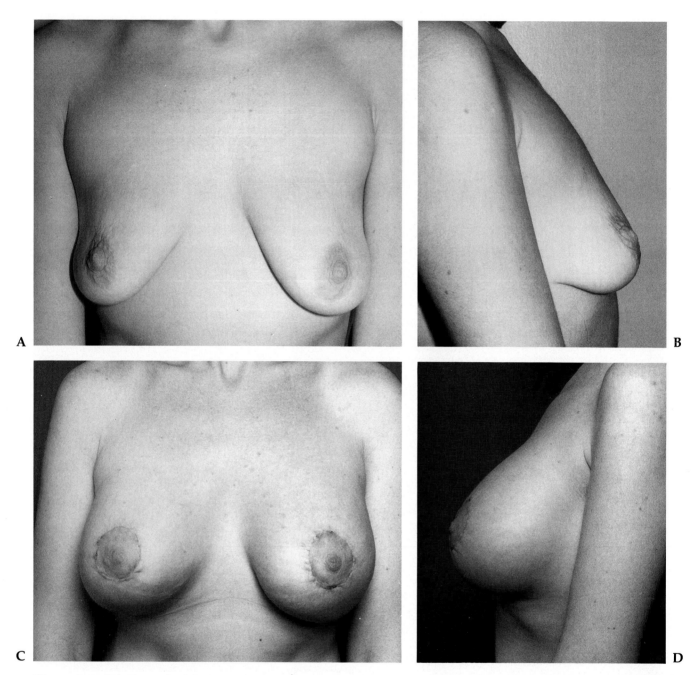

Figure 8.9. (A) Frontal and **(B)** lateral preoperative views of a 36-year-old woman with breast ptosis and hypotrophy. **(C, D)** Postoperative appearance after circumareolar mammoplasty and breast implantation: **(C)** frontal; **(D)** lateral.

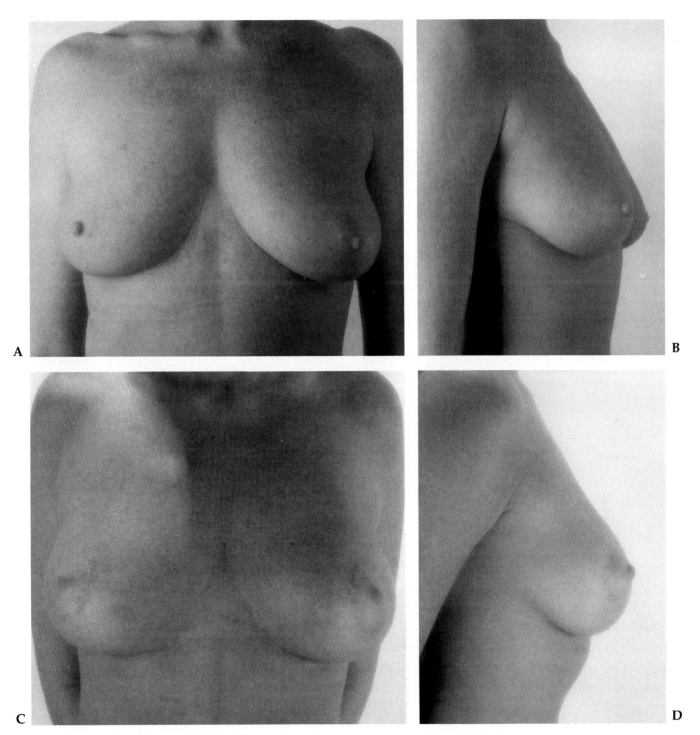

Figure 8.10. **(A)** Frontal and **(B)** lateral preoperative views of a 39-year-old woman with breast ptosis. **(C, D)** Postoperative appearance after circumareolar mammoplasty: **(C)** frontal; **(D)** lateral.

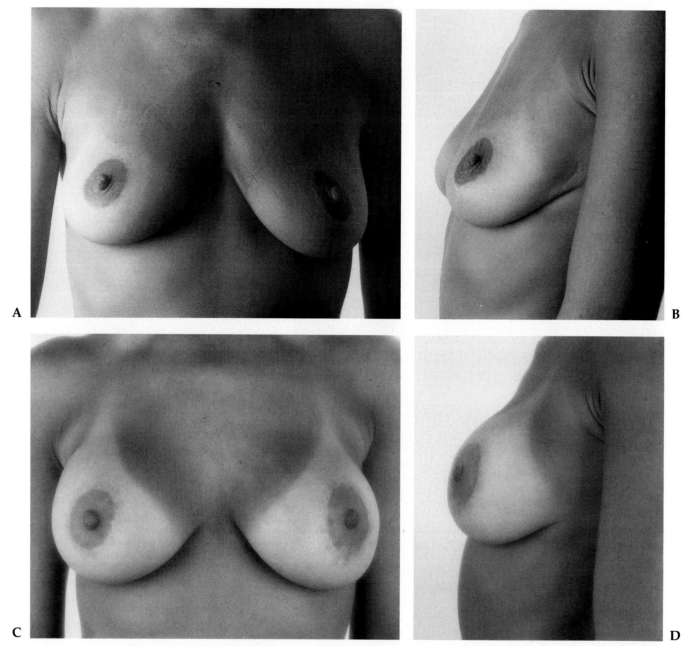

Figure 8.11. **(A)** Frontal and **(B)** lateral preoperative views of a 33-year-old woman with breast underdevelopment and ptosis. **(C, D)** Postoperative condition after breast implantation and circumareolar mammoplasty: **(C)** frontal; **(D)** lateral.

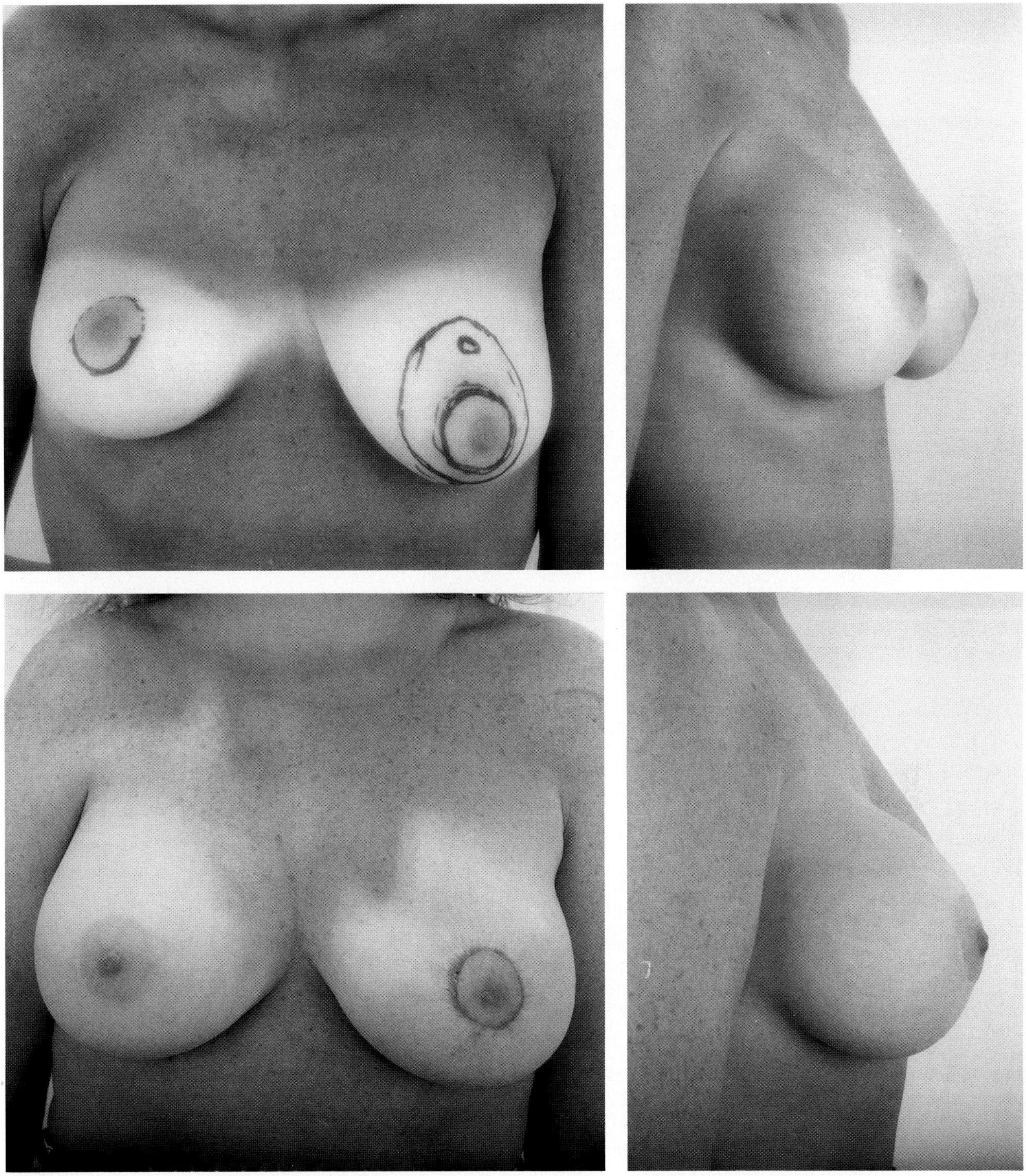

Figure 8.12. (A) Frontal and **(B)** lateral preoperative views of a 26-year-old woman with uneven breasts with ptosis and underdevelopment. **(C, D)** Postoperative appearance after right breast implantation through a periareolar incision and left breast implant with circumareolar mammoplasty: **(C)** frontal; **(D)** lateral.

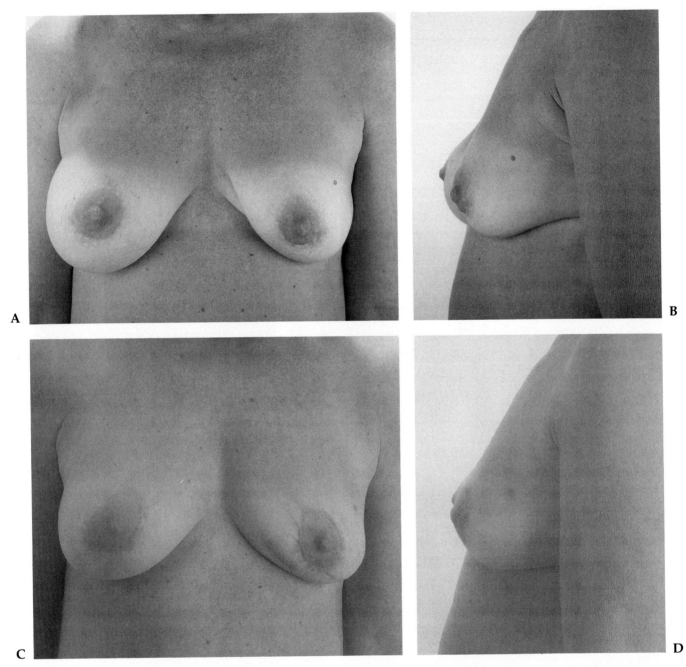

Figure 8.13. **(A)** Frontal and **(B)** lateral preoperative views of a 36-year-old woman with right breast implant and ptosis and left breast ptosis. (The implant extruded spontaneously after infection 5 years after implantation on the left side.) **(C, D)** Postoperative appearance after removal of the right implant and circumareolar mammoplasty: **(C)** frontal; **(D)** lateral.

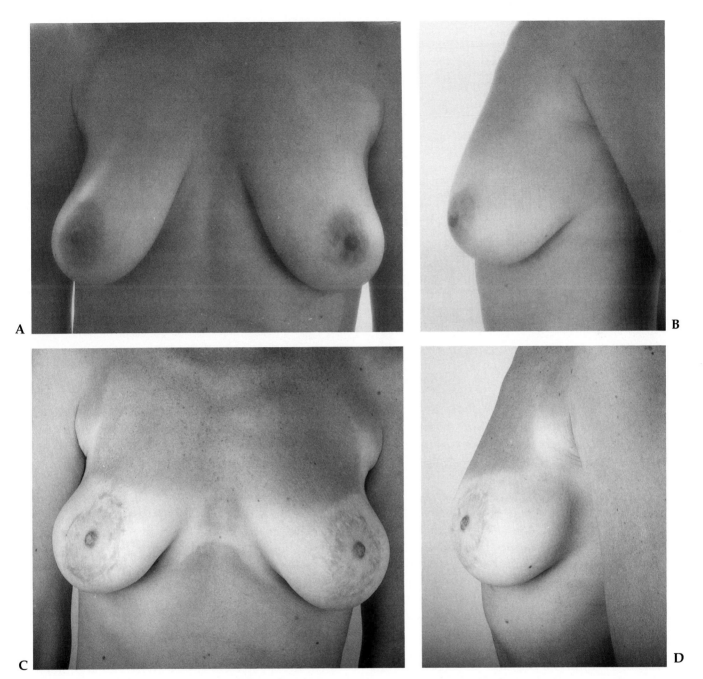

Figure 8.14. **(A)** Frontal and **(B)** lateral preoperative views of a 40-year-old woman with breast ptosis and hypotrophy. **(C, D)** Postoperative appearance after circumareolar mammoplasty: **(C)** frontal; **(D)** lateral.

Comments

Luiz S. Toledo

The Brazilian techniques of Arié, Pitanguy, and Peixoto can be used not only for mastopexy, but also for the reduction of large, moderate, and small breast hypertrophies.

Arié's[1] breast reduction technique, dating from 1957, resects gland in a lozenge shape and leaves a vertical scar that crosses the inframammary fold. The technique has not been used for breast reduction after the bikini became popular, but many of the vertical incision mammoplasty techniques used today are based in Arié's principles.

Pitanguy[2] substituted for Arié's lozenge shape a keel-shaped gland resection, transforming the vertical scar to an inverted T, and keeping all the incisions within the brassiere-covered area. This allowed for good reduction and shape improvement, while maintaining the integrity of breast function. The main advantage of the Pitanguy technique is that skin and gland resection is performed en bloc, without skin dissection, and thus there is no dead space.

Peixoto's[3] technique uses smaller incisions and resects gland from the base of the mammary cone, removing less skin and counting on skin retraction to obtain the final shape of the breast.

In Figures 8.7 through 8.14, Adrien Aiache shows cases of mastopexy, breast reduction, and augmentation. Although the periareolar incision approach is the same, these are three different procedures. Flatness of the upper pole is more difficult to avoid in reduction than in augmentation, and scar stretching and areolar enlargement should be less of a problem in reduction than in augmentation.

References
1. Arié G: Una nueva técnica de mastoplastia. Rev Latinoamericana Cir Plast 3:23, 1957.
2. Pitanguy, I: Mammaplastias estudo de 245 casos consecutivos apresentaçao de tecnica pessoal. Rev Br Cir 42:20, 1961.
3. Peixoto, G: Reduction mammaplasty: A personal technique. Plast Reconstr Surg 65:217, 1980.

Techniques for Reduction of Larger Breasts

Tolbert S. Wilkinson

As discussed earlier, circumareolar surgery was initially performed only for smaller mastopexies; in time its use gradually expanded to include smaller and moderate size breast reductions. Steps were taken to prevent an ultimately flat ("pancake") appearance, as well as areolar expansion. This is particularly important in large breast reduction, because the swelling of the tissues following the reduction puts extra pressure on the areola-skin junction.

My method of breast reduction is essentially a subcutaneous Pitanguy wedge with resetting of the mammary mound at a higher position. During the presentation of our teaching course at the annual meeting of the American Society for Plastic and Reconstructive Surgeons, Louis Benelli commented that he uses a superior pedicle technique with his circumareolar "round block" procedure. I believe the Pitanguy wedge, described in detail below, is probably safer, and certainly easier to create.

The addition of liposuction must be viewed with some concern. In the past year one of my patients suffered a partial areolar loss; this occurred on the side I had liposuctioned to reduce the bulk to match the opposite side. Although it is

possible that a hemorrhage occurred, because the change in areolar perfusion color became apparent by the twelfth hour postsurgery, it may be wise to defer liposuction for a later date in the patients with very large breasts who request a significant tissue mass reduction.

When describing the circumareolar reduction to my younger patients, I emphasize that the advantages outweigh the disadvantages. Since scars on the skin of the chest are even more unpredictable in younger than in older patients, and because clothing styles have changed (with patients having an aversion to scars far greater today than when I first entered practice), our patients are usually ready to accept a longer period of remodeling and healing in the periareolar area to avoid the discomfort and possible hypertrophy of the inferior and vertical scars of standard breast reduction.

There are certain patients in whom circumareolar mastopexy should not be considered. These include older patients, patients with poor-quality skin, and those impatient individuals who demand that the breast be "presentable" in a short period of time. For these individuals a standard breast reduction is employed. As shown in Fig-

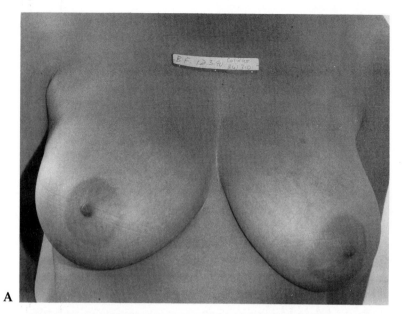

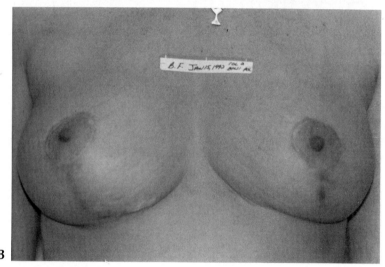

Figure 9.1. McKissock reduction. Because it is as easy to do a double pedicle as it is to do a superiorly or inferiorly based single pedicle, I prefer the security of the double pedicle procedure, particularly in patients such as this one. At this breast length, a free nipple graft is not the best choice. Neither is a circumareolar reduction because of the quality of the skin and the size of the circle that would require deepithelialization, although we are now approaching more of this category of patient **(A)** with the circle procedure. In **(B),** the excellent elevation of the areola is shown. Note, however, that even with careful multilayered approximation, thick scars are present in the circumareolar area at 2 years. Experiences such as this one have led me to apply the technique of "internal" reduction with the circumareolar technique to more patients with this degree of breast hypertrophy. If the best bipedicle reduction still requires "touch-up" surgery of the periareolar incision, why not avoid incisions elsewhere if one can obtain this degree of projection?

ures 9.1 and 9.2, I prefer a McKissock double pedicle technique, leaving a "thick" pedicle. This preserves a larger number of ducts. On the other hand, the circumareolar technique protects the ducts from injury because the reduction is a lower one-third wedge removal.

In older patients the decision must be made between standard reduction and free nipple grafting. Surprisingly, many authors have reported that patients recover sensation in free nipple grafts, and this has been my experience as well. Nevertheless, there remain the possibilities of loss of color and even loss of the graft. In many older patients, recovery of only a portion of

sensation is more than adequate; for them the breast is no longer a sexual organ and nipple sensation plays a lesser role in their lifestyle than in the younger patient. Free grafts, therefore, are less risky. The second of my two complications of partial nipple loss occurred 5 days following a circumareolar reduction in a young patient with an *extremely* long and ptotic breast. In an older patient I would have recommended free nipple grafting. The fact that the partial necrosis occurred after discharge from the hospital and may be attributed to compression or other outside factors is not important at this point; we must strive to make all procedures as complication free as possible. Fortunately, in younger patients, the remaining areola will expand after the debridement and it is easy enough to create a rounded nipple of 4 cm at the appropriate postoperative time.

Another argument for the circumareolar reduction technique in the younger patient is the relative security of the nerve supply, because the circumareolar area is deepithelialized only superficially. Our patients have recovered sensation in all cases to date. Preservation of the ducts for later breast feeding is a concern for many modern women. The circumareolar technique by the Pitanguy wedge procedure preserves most of the ductal system. In addition, ducts are not transsected when the nipple is lifted onto the mass of the breast as it is coned and moved upward.

The general principles of breast reduction for larger breasts are similar to those of mastopexy and smaller reductions. The measurements first are for a nipple position at the ideal level, some 18 to 19 cm from the sternal notch. When the areola is elevated (Toledo triangle or Texas diamond excision above the areola) the nipple is secure at this position. As noted in Chapter 1, I now make the nipple less than 4 cm because there is inevitably some expansion. A diameter of 3.8 cm seems to work best. The second measurement from areola to inframammary fold, is also the same as for mastopexy. Because of the greater length involved from the new areolar edge to the inframammary fold, one leaves additional skin length. In the classic McKissock procedure, one draws the lower limb to be 5 to 6 cm in length. No skin retraction is involved. In the circumareolar technique for large breasts the skin is undermined widely and will retract into the newly elevated inframammary fold, and will shrink as well. For this reason I leave a distance of 8 to 9 cm between the current inframammary fold and the lower edge of the circle. The two points are then joined with an estimate of the amount of skin that must be resected laterally and medially. This circle or oval is then deepithelialized.

As noted in Chapter 4, when freeing the breast skin, it is important to dissect in the subcutaneous tissue rather than beneath the dermis. The extra layer of fatty tissue provides a cushion for contour and protects the blood supply in the skin. Once the dissection is carried out to the inframammary fold it is continued medially until the area is reached where the breast begins to join into the sternum. This must be preserved so that the patient does not have an exaggerated separation of the new breasts. The lateral dissection can be carried out all the way to the nine o'clock position. After removing the Texas triangle and setting the areola, my assistant holds the breast skin away so that the Pitanguy excision can be carried out. This is not only a central wedge, which is varied according to the size, wishes, and requirements of the patient, but a lateral wedge at the inframammary fold to shorten the length of the inverted V. The limbs should be shortened to between 5 and 6 cm to create a proper cone. In contrast to the infolding or overlapping procedure required by other patients, the large breast reduction patient can be corrected by simple closure of the V in layers. Careful lateral liposuction, rather than the direct debulking performed in the McKissock or other pedicle procedures, is usually required.

The bottom points of the inverted V are joined and sutured to the underlying pectoralis fascia at an overcorrected position, usually some 2 to 3 cm above the original inframammary fold. Additional inverted and figure-eight sutures of #1 Vicryl continue the coning. Once it is complete, scissors are used to trim any surface irregularities so that a rounded, tall breast mound is left in its new elevated position. At this point we are ready to begin the circumareolar closure.

It is certainly more difficult to obtain a smoother contour in these larger patients and one is often tempted to take a "lollipop" wedge of skin. To test the limits of this procedure, I avoided this temptation in the cases that are presented. Taking the wedge will certainly ensure a quicker resolution of the crumpling, but I have found that it is not necessary in the long-term appearance of the nipple, areola, and surrounding skin. Larger breast reduction patients must be prepared to wait 6 to 18 months while this infolded tissue slowly resolves. When the closure is done as described in Chapters 3 and 4, care is taken that the majority of the folded tissue is placed in the lower part of the circle, between the five and seven o'clock positions. The weight

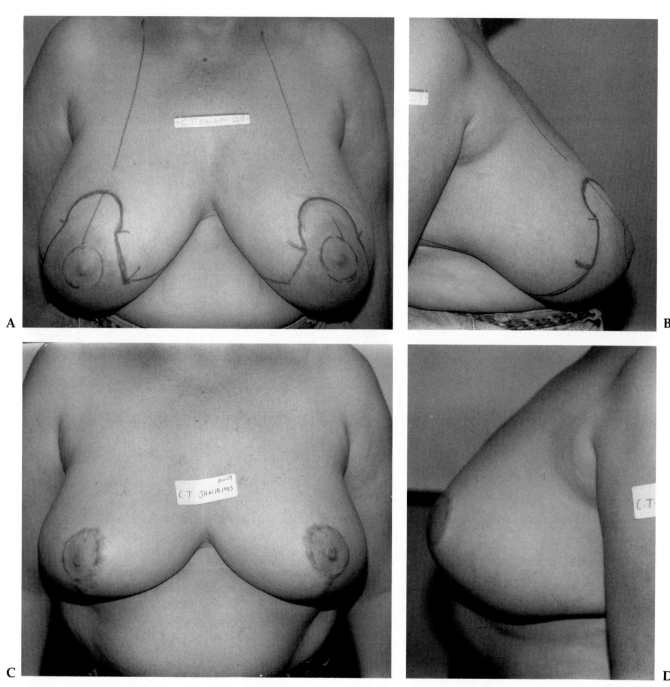

Figure 9.2. Standard reduction mammoplasty. The results for standard mastopexy are immediate, predictable, and quite satisfactory. For the younger patient, however, even the shortened horizontal scar as shown will be distressing. In this McKissock bipedicle reduction **(A, B),** the horizontal incisions were kept underneath the fold of the breast both medially and laterally. Unfortunately, this patient is typical in that the scars are still hypertrophic and angry in appear-ance, despite a regimen of skin care, topical steroids, and occasional scar injections. The circumareolar approach eliminates all but the scars in the center of the breast **(C, D),** an area of direct pressure from the brassiere **(E).** Pressure is important in controlling scar hypertrophy, yet it is our experience that the medial and lateral ends of the standard mastopexy scars often require scar revisions, and frequently multiple revisions until a more satisfactory appearance is obtained.

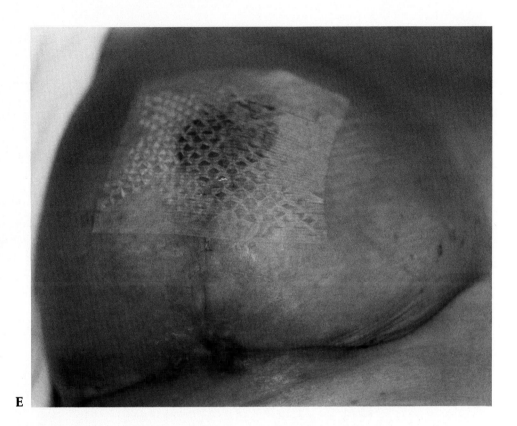

E

of the breasts against the brassiere acts as a pressure mechanism to hasten resolution in this area. It is also a less visible zone. Only a minimal amount of skin folding should be visible in the upper circle, between the ten o'clock and two o'clock positions.

As shown in Figure 9.3A, the wedge has been removed and the lateral limbs have been shortened in preparation for suturing. In Figure 9.3B one or two layers of inverted sutures have been placed in the midline and the anchoring sutures horizontally are holding the new cone in its elevated position.

Because of natural asymmetries and the vagaries of planning the degree of wedge to be excised, I have often found it necessary to reintroduce a 3-mm liposuction cannula, this time through the drain site, for further reduction on one side or another. As noted above, this must be done carefully. Drains are always necessary and these patients require continued postoperative support.

An example of moderate reduction of large breasts is described in Figure 9.4.

In closing the area around the areola in the McKissock or other "standard" breast reductions, I place a series of Dexon 4-0 sutures in the deep subcutaneous tissue to bring the edges together. Because there is no deepithelialized ring, a circle Benelli-type double suture is not necessary and would not help. Tacking stitches are used more frequently than with circle closures, and are usually of the half-buried variety tied loosely on the areolar skin. If a stitch mark should result, it mimicks the appearance of the Montgomery gland. There is still drainage from the edges, however, and the Mesh tape described in the caption to Figure 9.2E is useful. This tape may be applied 24 hr after the breast reduction to immobilize the skin and the areola and yet allow drainage into the overlying dressing. I commonly leave this tape in place for 10 to 12 days.

In 1969, when I was a resident in plastic surgery at St. Louis University (St. Louis, MO), I developed Mesh tape as a means of immobilizing skin grafts. With a grant from the 3M Company a commercial preparation of Mesh tape followed and it was made available to other surgeons for

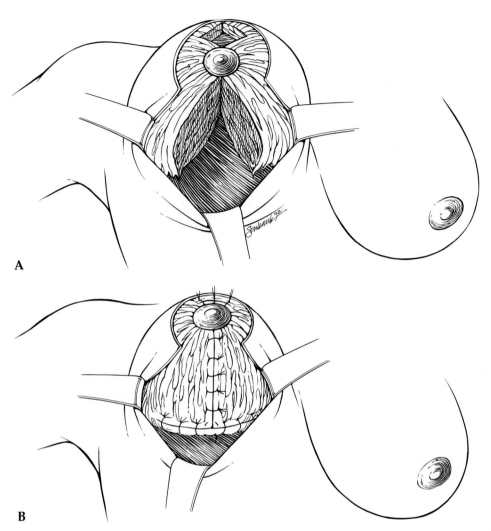

A

B

Figure 9.3. Reduction of the large breast is essentially the same as for the smaller breast. **(A)** The deepithe-lialized area is designed so that the nipple-areolar complex may be brought upward to its new position. This is only a partial-thickness soft tissue excision, leaving the majority of the blood supply intact over the upper two thirds of the breast. With the skin reflected, a Pitanguy wedge is excised. In **(B)**, the left and right sides have been trimmed to an appropriate length based on the position of the now secured nipple-areolar complex. This distance should measure 5 to 6 cm. Anchoring sutures are then used to secure the lower edges to the pectoralis fascia and a series of imbricating sutures are used to secure the cone shape beneath the skin.

Figure 9.4. Major breast reduction in an older patient. Fortunately, this patient requested that her breasts be reduced only moderately. Because of her large bone structure and perhaps as a response to her recent abdominoplasty and major liposuction of the lower body, she had requested that her breasts be left in a fairly large state. **(A)** Note the extreme width of the deepithe-ialization and the wide Texas diamond that will be removed from each areola. This patient's reduction was performed as a demonstration surgery under ketamine-diazepam (Valium) anesthesia. One error was made in that we did not drain and a seroma developed on the left side some 10 days postoperatively, resulting in extrusion of the Mersilene suture and a moderate amount of swelling medially. The patient was so pleased with the results **(B)** that she would not allow the final adjustment, which would include minor liposuction and a revision of the left-side scar.

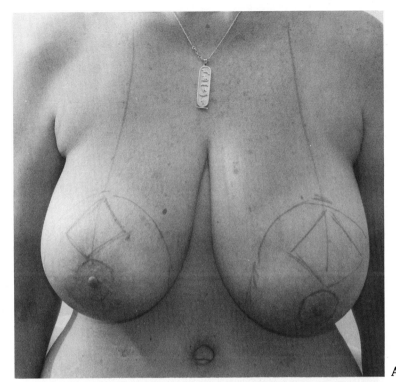

A

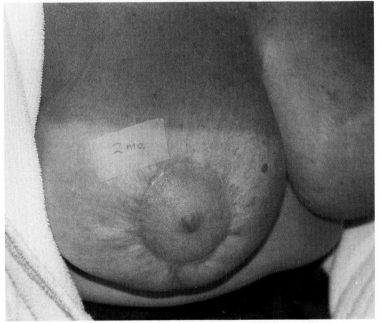

B

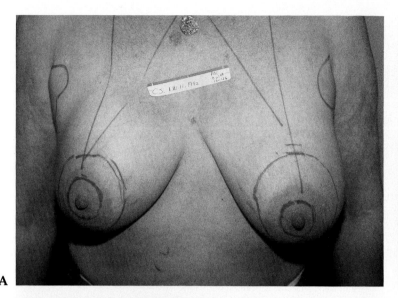

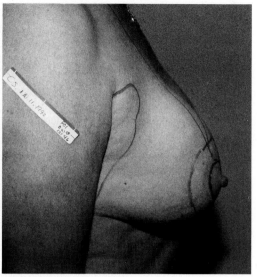

A

B

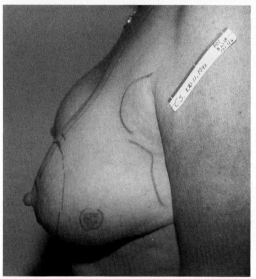

C

Figure 9.5. Markings for large breast reduction. See text for details.

mobilization of skin grafts and finger tip replacements, where it has proved its worth.

Markings for Larger Breast Reductions

The markings for breast reduction are essentially the same as for smaller reductions and mastopexy, with the addition of a marking for liposuction of the axilla and the area posterior to the anterior axillary line. As shown in Figure 9.5A–C, the initial measurements from the sternal notch and the midclavicle are made and then a visual

adjustment is considered. On this patient's left side this resulted in lowering the new nipple position below the measured position. Notice also the differences to account for asymmetry and that the areolar size has been reduced to less than 4.0 cm.

The second marking is made at a distance 9 cm from the inframammary fold in the midline. These points are then connected with either an ellipse, as shown on the patient's left (Figure 9.5C), or circle, as shown on the patient's right (Figure 9.5B). This is the area that will be deepithelialized. The distance between the top of the circle and the edge of the new areola will be

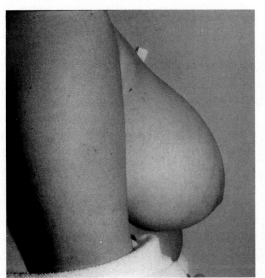
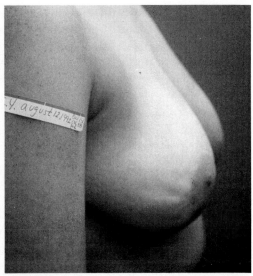

Figure 9.6. Moderate reduction of larger breasts, using the circumareolar technique. **(A, B)** Patient C.Y.; **(C, D)** patient C.S.

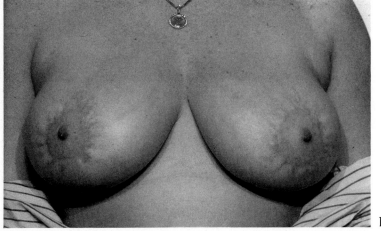
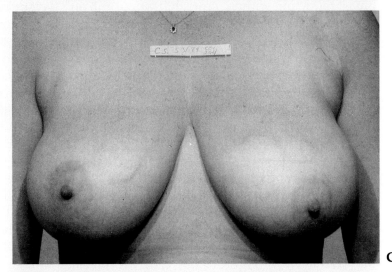

excised to a depth of 1 cm so that the new areola will be fixed at this preferred position. As described, I now make this nipple position exactly the same as would be selected for a McKissock or other pedicle flap reduction, because the danger of "star gazing" has not materialized in this series of circumareolar reductions.

Moderate Circumareolar Reductions in Young Women With Large Breasts

Our experience with large reductions, using the circumareolar technique, came as a result of requests from patients; these patients wanted breast reduction without scars that would rub on brassieres or bikini tops. Patients C.Y. and C.S. (Figure 9.6), who typify these patients, desired initially only a modest reduction in volume. Because their skin quality was excellent, I decided to try the circumareolar technique with only a moderate amount of liposuction adjustment (liposuction has made this technique even more effective).

Patient C.Y. is shown preoperatively in 1989 (Figure 9.6A) and 5 months postoperatively (Figure 9.6B). The shape conformed to her wishes for a modest reduction. We have received reports that the shape has remained the same and that the wrinkling has since disappeared. Notice in her lateral view (Figure 9.6B) that the breast retains a cone shape, from the internal wedge resection and cone formation with resetting of the inframammary fold. In this initial group of moderate circumareolar reductions, I was more concerned with subsequent areolar lifting to an unacceptable position and purposely placed the areola at a somewhat lower spot. Note the difference in patient C.S., who had a modest reduction in 1990 (Figure 9.6C and D), and for whom a higher areolar position was chosen (Figure 9.6D).

When Not to Use a Circumareolar Reduction

I am not comfortable with circumareolar reduction of massively enlarged breasts (e.g., Figure 9.7) or of breasts that have multiple stretch marks, which indicate a poor quality of skin retraction and dermal blood supply. In 1983, the patient L.S. (Figure 9.7) asked for a premarital breast reduction. At age 23, her breasts had reached a size that caused her considerable symptomatology. Notice the strap marks on her shoulders and the relative symmetry of the breast enlargement. We used a standard McKissock reduction and changed her to a small C cup. Nine years later, she presented with the problem shown in Figure 9.7F–G. Her breasts had continued to enlarge almost from the day of the operation. When this amount of tissue has regenerated, it is advisable to remove the nipple and replace it as a free nipple graft, and completely remove the ductal system at the same time. This is not a 100% guarantee against recurrence of virginal hypertrophy but it certainly should reduce the risk. At 6 months, her breasts have retained the size and shape that we recreated. Note in the preoperative drawings (Figures 9.7D and E) that liposuction will be used in the anterior axillary line area. The long incision is placed to meet the original long incision from 1983. Today, we keep these incisions shorter, even in the larger patients, because the "dog ear" that is located beneath the breast fold will flatten nicely with time.

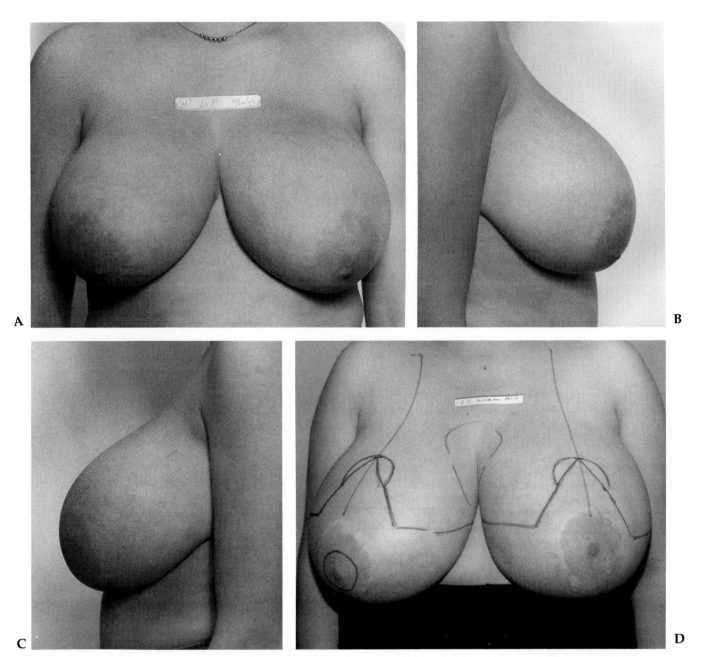

Figure 9.7. (A–C) Patient J.S. in 1988; her breasts were reduced using the standard McKissock technique. **(D–G)** The same patient in 1992. See text for details.

Figure 9.7. *Continued*

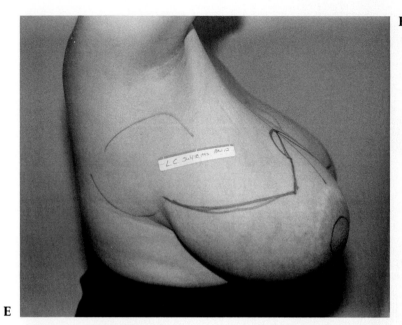

E

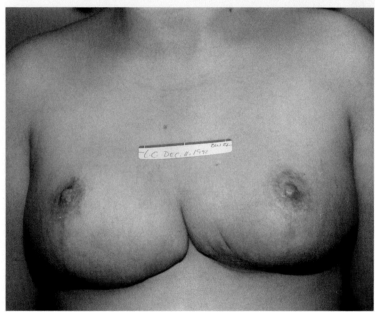

F

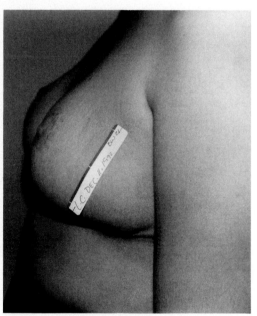

G

Comments

Adrien Aiache

Only rarely have I encountered a patient whose large breasts are amenable to reduction by circumareolar mastopexy. I usually feel that the excessive breast enlargement makes it difficult to obtain the double advantage of relatively satisfactory breast reduction associated with good shape and an acceptable scar. I would be tempted to reserve the circumareolar technique in large breast reduction to the patient who happens to have very loose skin. This allows her breasts to be reduced by liposuction more than by actual surgical reduction, thus easing the actual reduction and imposing less taxing demands on the tissues of the skin to hold the breast mound.

Comments

Luiz S. Toledo

One of the major qualities I find in Wilkinson's work is that, despite being widely known and a recognized expert in the field of breast surgery, he is still interested in trying new techniques and enhancing his own skills by their incorporation, should they prove worthy. As one of the pioneers in the periareolar approach, Wilkinson has constantly searched for new ways to improve his results, as can be seen in this chapter, in which he reveals his sources and what has influenced him. This is a clear, "how to" chapter for both the expert and the beginner wanting to perform this procedure.

✢ 10 ✢

Repair: Adapting Circumareolar Techniques to Breast Repair Surgery

Tolbert S. Wilkinson

Adapting the circumareolar principles for repair of the distorted or stretched breast is valuable for the practicing surgeon. Either from low placement of a breast prosthesis, or from stretching due to gravitational or muscular factors, a number of patients are presenting us with the problem of ballooning of the lower half of the breast with or without areolar descent. The principles of "subcutaneous mastopexy" are used to recreate the original shape of the breast with restoration of the inframammary fold position and with the reinforcement of the thinned parenchyma. The cross-over procedure is a deterrent to future ptosis of this area, and the entire repair is performed by way of the original short periareolar augmentation incision. The idea of repositioning the nipple-areolar complex without a vertical or horizontal scar was intriguing enough for many of us to try this operation for patients who needed reparative surgery. The patient in Figure 10.1A was one of these cases. She had requested a small breast augmentation in 1979 to fill out the upper quadrant. By 1992 the lower half of her breasts had stretched, and the nipples had dropped to a lower position as well. The original periareolar

incision was used for implant replacement and internal repair. There was no deepithelialization and no circular suture, and of course no liposuction for balancing. With the skin reflected I was able to do a very thick multilayered closure from the vertical splitting incision that allowed me to create the pocket.

As the years passed, this patient continued to do well, and began to show the changes shown in Figure 10.1D, E, F only after 2 years. In similar, more recent cases performed without the internal tightening and areolar lift, I have often noted greater degrees of descent than shown by these early patients. Others typically had a very slow descent, probably owing to the fibrosis in the vertical repair. In retrospect, the scarring around the areolae is not as acceptable by today's standards, but I must point out that this type of blurred scar was typical of our standard breast reductions in 1979, using the anchor scar. This patient illustrates the advantages of the periareolar elevation with the addition of infolding and tightening in the most vulnerable area, the stretchable tissue between the areola and the inframammary fold.

147

Figure 10.1

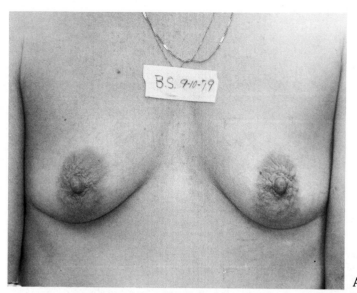

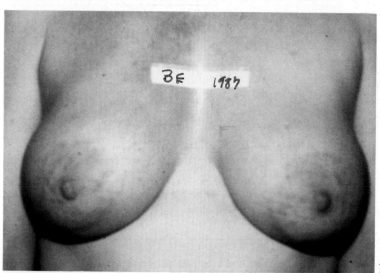

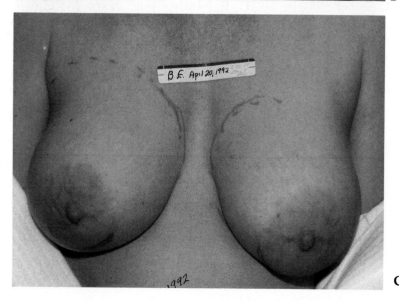

D

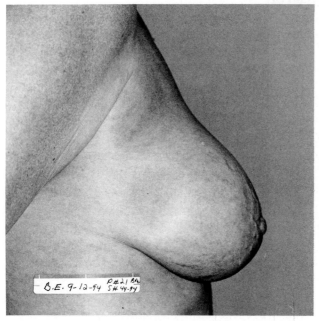

E

F

Figure 10.1. Patient BS is pictured in **(A)** in her preoperative state following pregnancy. There is a minimal amount of asymmetry, one would not expect the slow descent, particularly on the left side, that occurred. This was evident to a minor degree in her 1987 photograph **(B)**. By 1992, the inevitable effect of gravity and age resulted in a marked asymmetry, particularly with descent on the left side **(C)**. Using the principles of internal repair, the short periareolar incisions were utilized and a new prosthesis of the textured type was positioned at a higher spot. The excess tissue length between the areolar and the new inframammary fold was resected, and then a left-to-right overlapping reinforcement was carried out on both sides with a greater degree of elevation on the left. Photographs taken at $2\frac{1}{2}$ years following the internal repair **(D, E, F)** show that the internal repair has maintained breast position and an acceptable mildly ptotic shape that is consistent with her age, lifestyle, and personal wishes.

Postpartum Ptosis With Breast Prostheses

Most American patients with breast prostheses who experience postpartum ptosis want their breasts restored to their original shape, along with the fullness they once enjoyed. In these cases it is important to remember that this stretched skin will contract. The markings for these patients are illustrated in Figure 10.2A. In this patient areolar repositioning and areolar reduction are required. I now make a 3.8-cm circle around the nipple (not 4.2 cm) and, as noted above, make the top of the marking circle at the position to which this areola will be moved. In patients with this degree of ptosis it is necessary to remove skin both medially and laterally. These markings are done only after the six o'clock mark is placed. Remember that this skin will contract once the cone is established. This distance (inframammary fold to areolar edge) is left at 9 cm. The two points are then connected in an elliptical manner, as shown in Figure 10.2A, so that one may deepithelialize and reduce the distances between the new nipple and the sternum and lateral axillary lines.

It is also important to ascertain whether these patients request a smaller, higher, lifted breast or a more "mature" ptotic breast. The latter, of course, is easier to obtain in these patients and this is the shape and size to which they are accustomed. This reduces the need for a wide deepithelialization, thus reducing the time required for flattening of the areolar purse-string folds.

The greatest application of the internal mastopexy procedures is in the patient with postpartum or non-support-induced breast stretch following breast augmentation. These patients fall into two categories. The most common is the patient with "stretch out" from the areola to the inframammary fold without areolar descent. Correction involves the same principle of detachment of skin and in subcutaneous tissue from the lower half of the breast, but through a short periareolar incision. This also allows access to the overstretched zone. Vertical splitting of the breast is followed by resection of the excessive length at the inframammary fold level. Left and right flaps of breast tissue are designed and then folded one on the other; and a new and higher inframammary fold (Figure 10.2B) is established with absorbable polyglycolic sutures. Compression brassieres hasten realignment of the overly stretched skin in the lower half of the breast.

A complete circumareolar technique is used for the second type of postpartum stretching, which involves lower half stretch, areolar descent, and widening of the areola. An appropriate circle of areolar skin is deepithelialized. Once the inferior half skin and subcutaneous tissue has been retracted, the cross-over flaps for the identical treatment of the excess soft tissue are designed. Skin resection is not necessary in these patients (Figure 10.2C–E). The reinforcement of the inferior half of the breast parenchyma by the overlapping flaps appears to be retarding further descent in the majority of our cases, who have been followed for 5 years. Those followed for over 10 years show the same degree of stability.

Implant Replacement and Internal Flap Repair

In certain cases a more aggressive internal repair is indicated. These are patients whose breasts have thinned in one area, which leaves an unsightly appearance. I have encountered this problem in patients with saline implants, as well as in patients such as H.D. (Figure 10.3A and B), who had standard gel prostheses placed in 1979. Preoperative evaluation revealed that the original breast prostheses were quite small and separated, and heavily encapsulated. This was a common problem in 1979. We proceeded with a complete capsulectomy and replacement with a softer gel prosthesis, little suspecting that these implants might wear through or disintegrate in the next 10 years. This is exactly what occurred with this patient.

In my chapter "Internal Repair of the Breast" (*Symposium on Aesthetic Surgery of the Breast*, Vol. 44. Owsley JQ, Peterson RA [Eds.]. C. V. Mosby, St. Louis, 1978, pp. 312–325), I discussed a number of local flaps of muscle or capsule (Figure 10.4) that were required to repair breasts of the

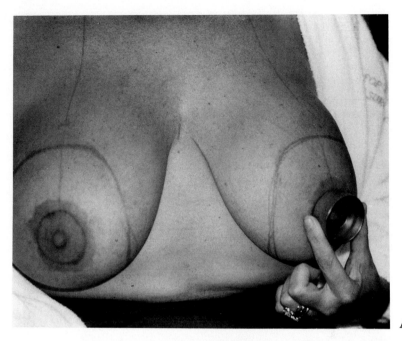

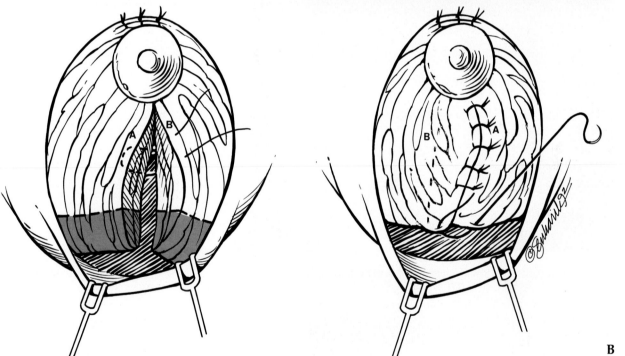

Figure 10.2. See text for details.

Figure 10.2. *Continued*

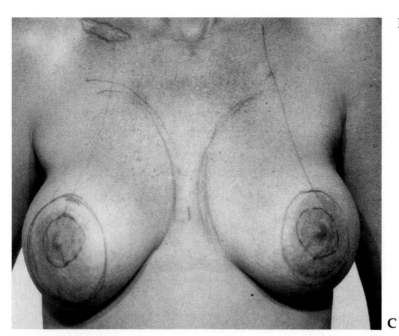

C

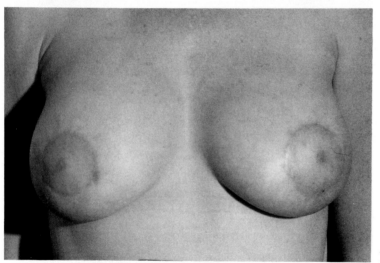

D

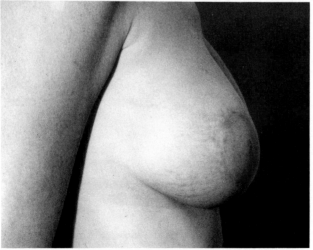

E

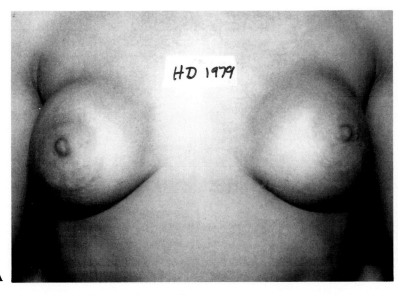
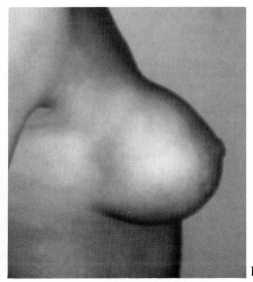

A

B

Figure 10.3. See text for details.

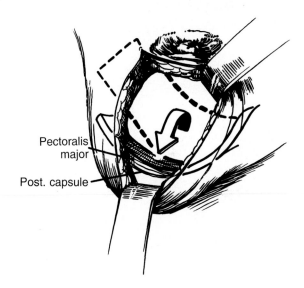

Pectoralis major

Post. capsule

Figure 10.4. See text for details.

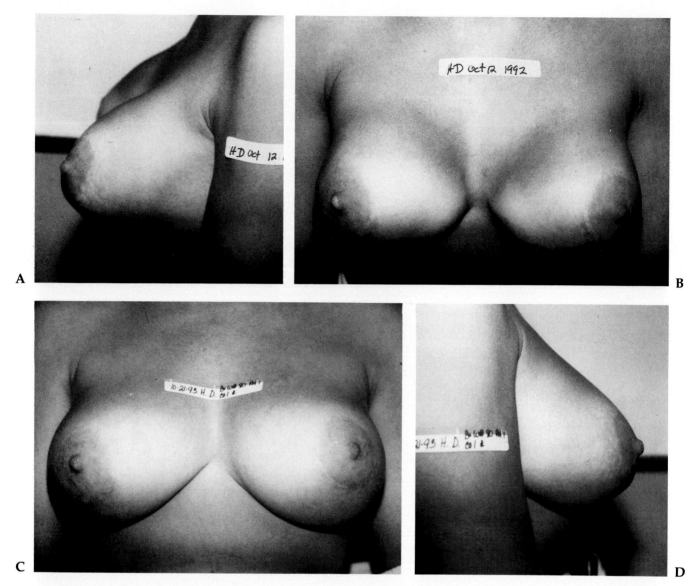

Figure 10.5. See text for details.

1970 augmentation era. These people often had overstretched zones, simply due to our aggressive use of steroids either into the dissected pocket or within the outer lumen of double prostheses. Patient H.D. developed a stretched area medially as well as breast descent.

Experience has taught that it is not sufficient simply to suture the capsule when medial overstretching has occurred (Figures 10.5A and B). I therefore approached this patient as a multiple internal repair candidate. We chose a wider-based textured prosthesis, which was positioned through her original small periareolar incisions.

An internal flap of pectoralis muscle and capsule based medially was turned upward on both sides and sutured into the defect. Capsulectomies were carried out in other areas and the capsule was fully expanded. Entry into the capsule was obtained through a vertical splitting incision to allow internal repair of the overstretched lower half. Notice in Figures 10.5C and D, taken 1 year following repair, that the curvature between the nipple and the inframammary fold has been restored and that the nipple appears to sit at a higher position with a greater degree of symmetry than was present in her original configura-

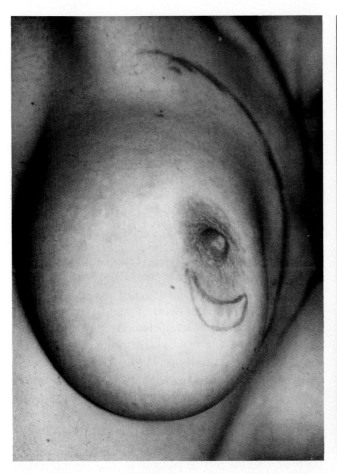

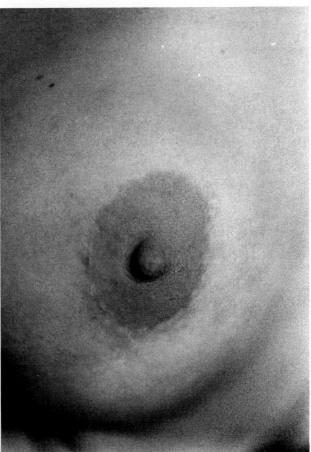

Figure 10.6. Deepithelialization of a small circle of skin.

Figure 10.7. A half-circle incision for full visualization.

tion. Removing the thickened capsule superiorally and laterally, and restoring and reinforcing the integrity of the breast wall between the three and nine o'clock positions, was as important in this patient as the internal rotation flaps that sealed off the medial overstretch.

Minimizing the Visibility of the Short Periareolar Incision

Patients who have had a periareolar incision are ideal for breast repair because full visualization of the stretched area is easily accomplished through this opening. Typically, the soft tissue has stretched in these patients. A small ellipse of skin may be deepithelialized, as shown in Figure 10.6. This deepithelialized area is used for further

reinforcement of the skin incision but skin removal is not required in the majority of cases.

Full visualization frequently requires a half-circle incision, as shown in Figure 10.7, but if closed well, it too will be acceptable. The first step is to close the deep subcutaneous shelf of soft tissue (Figure 10.8, top). The deeper tissues have been closed over the prosthesis. The skin and subcutaneous tissue are then advanced upward and secured by interrupted absorbable sutures (Dexon 4-0) at the deepest level of the subdermis (Figure 10.8). At this point I place an inverted vertical 4-0 suture in the deepest dermis and just above this a series of horizontal Dexon 4-0 sutures to bring the dermal tissue together. This gives an eversion of the skin edges. The final securing of this eversion is with a running subcuticular Dexon 5-0 suture with the end knot exteri-

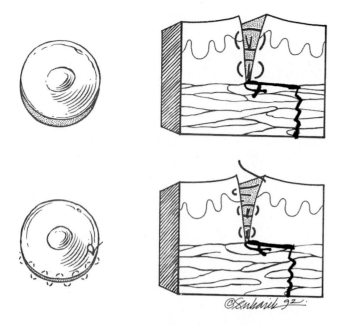

Figure 10.8. Diagram outlining closure of the deep subcutaneous shelf of soft tissue (bottom), and of the skin and subcutaneous tissue (top).

orized. The result is a scar that blends well into the junction between the pigmented areolar skin and the less pigmented breast skin (Figure 10.9). No surface tacking sutures are required. Skin tape support is used for 2 to 3 weeks following surgery.

Protecting the Microareola

In similar cases we have been faced with the problem of a very small areola, and yet I am reluctant to make an additional incision for the repair. I use a technique illustrated in Figure 10.10A and B. The first marking in Figure 10.10A shows the edge of the visible pigmentation at the areola. The second is a ring that will be deepithelialized. When tension is used to make the exposure for the internal repair there is no damage to the remaining tissue. This deepithelialized ring is also used for an advancing suture so that there is no tension on the closure, as shown in Figure 10.10B.

Internal Reinforcement

Once the chest wall has been exposed, several retractors are placed to elevate the skin as well as the breast tissue (Figure 10.11A). A scalpel is used for the initial cut-through, to save time, and then I change to an electric cautery to enter the capsule. At this point it is easy to free additional lateral tissue for visualization.

The left-to-right closure is also much easier at this point. Notice the curved retractor (Figure 10.11B) that holds the prosthesis away from the closure. The first suture is being placed on the undersurface laterally, so that the medial flap held in the forceps may be brought underneath and anchored to the undersurface. After placing a series of these sutures, the lateral flap is then brought over the medial and sutured to the outer surface of the breast wall. It is surprising how easy this is to carry out. Once one is familiar with the procedure a simple shifting of the retractors allows full visualization. When the final suture has been placed in the horizontal inframammary fold the protective retractor is simply slipped out and the last suture placed above.

Notice in the final sutures that the skin edges are already everted before the final securing suture of Dexon 5-0 is placed in the subcuticular tissue.

In internal repair in which the nipple-areolar complex has descended, the circle deepithelialization is carried out and a similar left-to-right closure is designed.

Ptosis Without Pregnancy

It is not unusual to see long-term breast augmentation patients with either lateral drift or unilateral ptosis due to the effect of gravity. Experienced surgeons are aware that breasts do not match in size, shape, nipple position, or in consistency. The latter contributes to the gravitational effect that not only may move the nipple downward, but stretches the lower portion of the breast between the nipple and the inframammary fold. In certain cases, such as the one shown in Figure 10.12A–C, nipple descent is a minor com-

Figure 10.9. The final result: the skin edges are everted, and the resulting scar will blend well with the surrounding tissues.

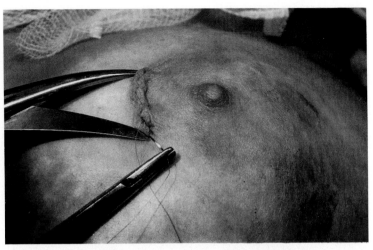

Figure 10.10. Protecting the microareola. See text for details.

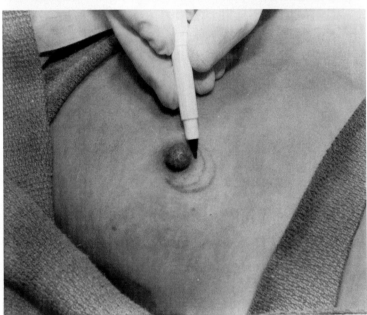

A

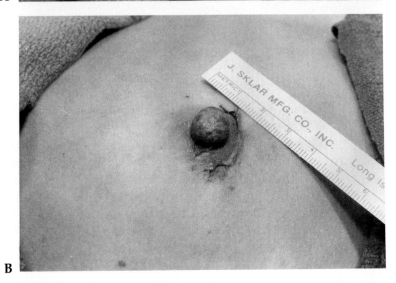

B

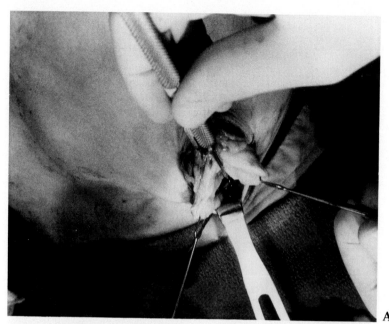

A

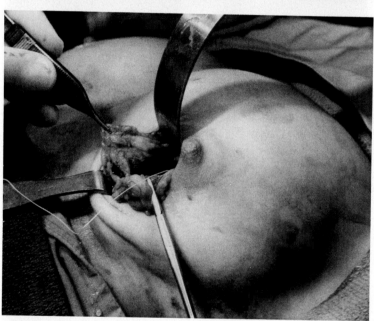

B

Figure 10.11. See text for details.

ponent. The internal repositioning and repair not only restored the contour for the next 10 years, but gave the illusion of nipple repositioning.

Figure 10.12A shows patient D.B. in 1984, several years following her breast augmentation. She had no history of trauma or pregnancy but admitted that the left breast had been descending for a number of years. When we discussed the changes she also requested that we increase the diameter and use a newer prosthesis, and this was accomplished. On the left side the entry was

made through the original periareolar incision. As we have often stated, the internal repair is technically more complex. In this case the complete circle incision was not required. Scar quality is satisfactory because of the shortness of the incision. As is our practice, this patient was operated on with ketamine-diazepam (Valium) dissociative anesthesia.

When the "dissociative" ketamine effect had been achieved, local anesthesia was used to infiltrate the lower half of the breast as well as to place

Figure 10.12. See text for details.

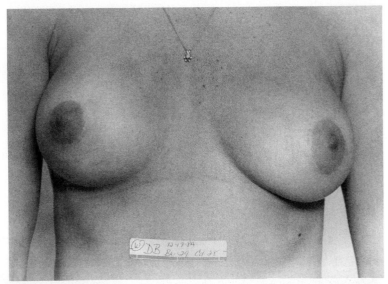

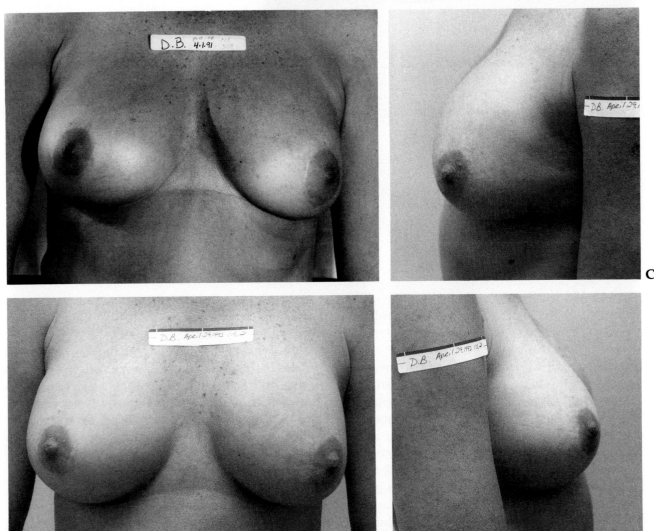

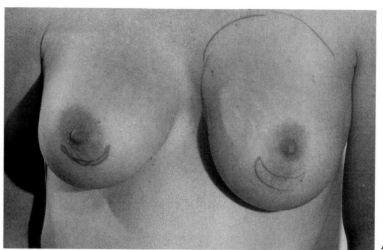

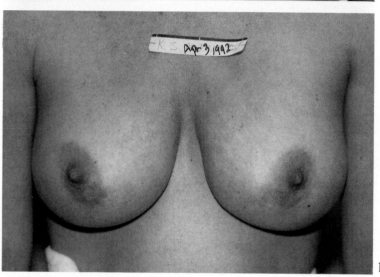

Figure 10.13. See text for details.

a field block. Once the lower skin had been reflected between the four o'clock and seven o'clock positions, a dissection that extends beyond the exposure afforded by the short incision, a vertical split was made in the breast wall. The capsule in this case was found to be normal (this is the usual finding). Once the new implant had been positioned, a small wedge was resected to shorten the distance between the nipple and the inframammary fold. In this case the inframammary fold had not descended. The left-to-right cross-over was accomplished using heavy absorbable sutures, first setting the left flap to the undersurface of the right. After this had been secured the right flap was then secured with

sutures to the outer surface of the opposite side and tacking stitches were placed in the horizontal component.

In these cases, the usual multilayered closure is carried out. The remaining Dexon 2-0 sutures were used to place one advancing suture into the deep dermis and to the breast wall 1 cm below the incision. Inverted Dexon 4-0 sutures have been used at intervals, and then horizontal Dexon 4-0 sutures are placed until the skin edges evert without tension. I end this closure with a subcuticular Dexon 5-0 suture, bringing the final loop knot through the skin for later removal.

As noted in her 1991 and 1993 photographs (Figure 10.12B–E), 10 years following the repair, there has been little change in the position or shape of the breast, presumably due to the double reinforcing sutures.

When a patient presents with an overstretched breast, such as patient K.S. in Figure 10.13A, one must assume that the condition existed prior to another surgeon's breast augmentation. There can be an unusual reason for overstretch, however. Mammograms on this patient showed a "bubble" adjacent to the prosthesis. It was read as a break in the prosthesis. What we found explained the ptosis as well as the usual mammogram appearance. The original surgeon had made a periareolar incision, but had dissected partially under the pectoralis muscle! When he inserted the implant, one third of the prosthesis was folded under the muscle and the remaining portion was trapped in the lower part of the breast, adding to the ptotic appearance.

After discussing several options we jointly decided on a fuller profile and to do an internal repair on the left side (expecting, of course, to find a broken prosthesis). Our initial approach on the left was through the periareolar incision with a wide subcutaneous dissection so that the entire lower third of the breast wall could be visualized. A vertical splitting incision was done and the implant pocket exposed. After opening it with cautery, the position of the implant was discovered and it was removed. A larger-sized textured prosthesis was prepared for reinsertion. The length between the inframammary fold and the edge of the areola was shortened by 2 cm with a simple tissue resection. The textured prosthesis was placed in the expanded pocket superiorly and then the "left-to-right" reinforcement sutures were placed. This set her new inframammary fold at a higher position, shortened the nipple-to-inframammary fold distance, and provided a double reinforcement that keeps the

prosthesis at a higher position. She has maintained this shape for $2\frac{1}{2}$ years and is pleased with the symmetry obtained by the internal repair (Figure 10.13B).

Internal Repair of a Vertical Split Using "Internal Mastopexy" Techniques

This patient presented a dilemma. She had severe capsular contractures after saline prostheses had been implanted in another state through fairly large inframammary incisions. During a closed release, she had suffered a rupture of the left breast internally so that the prosthesis was palpable in a defect extending from the inferior margin of the areola halfway to her shoulder. This defect measured two finger breadths (Figure 10.14A–C). She adamantly refused visible incisions.

Correction was by bilateral implant replacement through periareolar incisions. This allowed us to expose the entire overstretched portion of the left breast so that a reinforcing closure could be effected. A modification of the circumareolar technique was employed. The central zone from the edge of the areola to the inframammary fold was incised as a superiorly based flap (Figure 10.14D). The flap was turned on itself and sutured into the defect of the breast, filling it completely. Once the new prosthesis was in place, the anterior wall repair was carried out and the inframammary fold repositioned to match the right side.

With a minimal incision, we were able to achieve a relative symmetry is her dissimilar breasts, to repair the defect in the upper portion of the left breast, and to repair the overstretch on the left and right sides with internal reinforcement (Figure 10.14E–G).

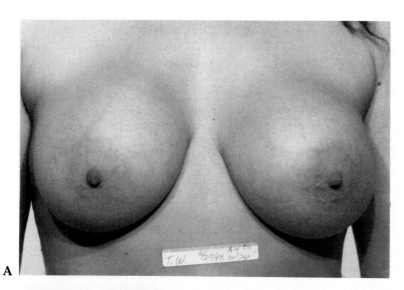

A

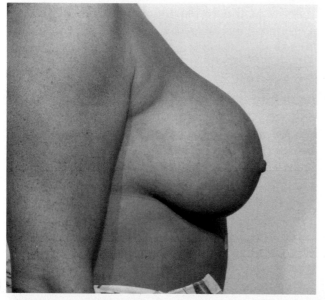

B

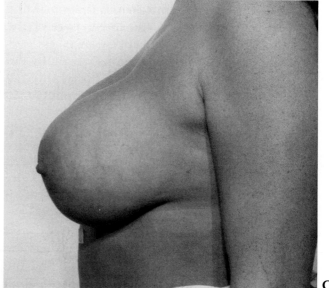

C

Figure 10.14. See text for details.

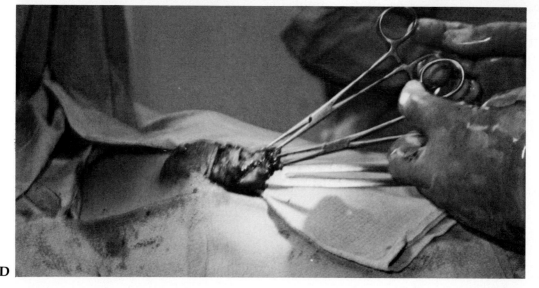

D

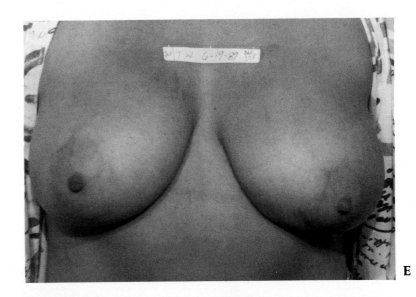

E

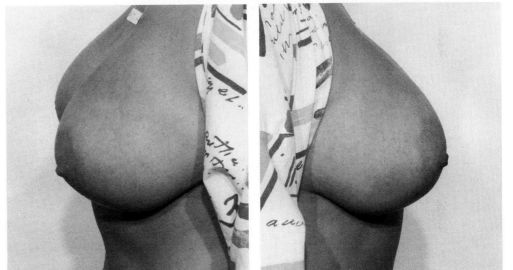

F

G

Circumareolar Mastopexy With Implant Removal or Replacement

Tolbert S. Wilkinson

Introduction

Five years ago, surgeons rarely saw patients who requested breast implant removal. There were many cases of replacement for increase or decrease in volume, and cases such as those described in Chapter 10 in which the breast had succumbed to gravitational forces and required some form of mastopexy or internal repair. Today, patients are requesting implant removal for good reasons (broken prostheses; siliconoma formation; slow increase in breast density and volume, making the implant unnecessary) or because they have been frightened by the flood of misinformation from activist groups and attorneys who are pursuing the theory that silicone breast implants cause systemic disease.

First, we physicians understand that this is not a silicone issue. It is a manufacturer liability issue confined to only one of many silicone devices. Science has little to do with the advice that our patients receive.[1-3] Patients receive silicone into their systems from their first "baby shot" to their last cup of coffee. We know that silicone sprays are used on fresh fruits and vegetables, ice cubes, coffee beans, and other items that we ingest. We know that silicone is inhaled when it is used in hairsprays. We know that all syringes and intra-

venous lines, blood transfusion bags, sutures, and so forth are coated in liquid silicone for good medical reasons. I tell my patients that anesthesiologists put more silicone into people than plastic surgeons do! Silicone was invented in the 1940s. It proved its value medically in neurosurgery with shunts to relieve intracranial pressure. Silicone is now an integral part of shunts in intraabdominal surgery, pacemakers, artificial joints, testicular and penile prostheses, ocular lenses, and other medical devices, even nipples on baby bottles. When I discuss the safety of medical devices with patients, I comment that *no* medical device or medication is 100% safe. If pacemakers were held to the same standards that are now proposed for silicone breast implants, there would be no pacemakers. There would also be very few drugs in use, from aspirin to penicillin.

We plastic surgeons must rely on experts in immunology, cancer research, and epidemiology to tell us what is correct information and what is not. As of 1994, we have no true scientific evidence of a direct linkage between inhaled, ingested, or injected silicone, or silicone in breast prostheses, and systemic disease. No one can identify antibodies to silicone. We are well aware that foreign body reactions occur with the breakdown of gel silicone and injected liquid silicone. The American Medical Association, the American College of Pathology, and the American Society of Rheumatology have issued statements condemning the hysteria and the "tests" that indicated the presence of inflammatory reaction only in patients with symptoms. Epidemiological studies from major universities in the United States and Europe were reported in 1993 and 1994.[4,5] The most important to plastic surgeons was the Los Angeles study[6] that has been ongoing for 15 years. This study logged 37,000 years of exposure to breast implants and compared two groups of women, those with implants and those without, to answer allegations that silicone causes breast cancer. The question had been raised because one species, among a number of laboratory animal species bred to develop tumors, did develop tumors when solid silicone balls were placed in their bodies. These animals also developed tumors of the sarcoma type when balls of glass, steel, or other materials were used. Humans do not do this. We were relieved, nonetheless, to learn that in the two Los Angeles groups, there were 48 cases of breast cancer in the group of women without implants and only 32 in the breast implant group. This may indicate a lesser incidence of carcinoma in smaller-breasted women. It reinforced the advice we have often given our breast augmentation patients. With good self-examinations, they are able to detect smaller lumps and the breast cancers that are detected should be in earlier stages. This has been the case in my practice and was the case in the cancers detected in the Los Angeles study.

It is distressing to hear knowledgeable physicians refer to "silicone-induced immune disease," when the only evidence that we have is that foreign body reactions occur to all medical devices, including breast implants. Reference is made in the lay press to Dow-Corning studies that showed a form of silicone inducing an immune response, but this contrived laboratory study involved materials that have never seen the inside of a human being. Antibodies that are identified in breast capsules appear to be the same antibodies that occur with any foreign material from splinters to artificial hips.

If the epidemiological studies of the immune response surveys, surveys of people with illegal silicone injections, surveys of patients with autoimmune disease that revealed that few, if any, had had breast implants, and other studies support our impression that silicone implants are not dangerous to the health, why would an implant be removed?

The answer is that there *were* physical problems with implants between 1970 and 1984. Documents discovered in malpractice actions against manufacturers revealed their concern with poorly constructed implants. Now we are aware that implants ruptured with minimal trauma, or even "self-destructed." We have also encountered implants that were composed of what appeared to be "motor oil," that is, liquid silicone that had not been converted into a solid gel. This silicone often produced an intense foreign body reaction.

In the past, it was unusual to see a patient with a broken prosthesis, and siliconomas were also rare; however, it was not unusual to see calcification in the capsules of the oldest implants. This interfered with self-examination and mammography. Beginning in 1989 we began to see patients with minimal trauma or no history of trauma whatsoever who had noted changes in their breasts. Good x-rays, physical examination, and subsequent surgery revealed broken prostheses with early intense inflammatory reaction in many cases. With these patients implant removal is a necessity.

Surgical Choices

If a patient requests implant removal for whatever reason, they are offered the choice between removal, replacement, and/or mastopexy. In the majority of these patients their breasts have descended. Fortunately, many of them have late developing breast hypertrophy that has occurred over 10 to 15 years. The techniques of circumareolar mastopexy are certainly applicable for these individuals and are illustrated below.

If a replacement prosthesis is not required or desired, why would one use circumareolar mastopexy rather than standard mastopexy? The most pressing reason is that these patients are already frightened and angry and the presence of additional scars after so many years without significant scarring is a concern. Even if a patient had an original incision in the inframammary fold, the majority of these scars are quiet and less conspicuous after 10 years. The circumareolar technique allows one to reposition all of the breast tissue after capsulectomy for creation of a mound and what is often an acceptable, smaller sized breast. In some of my patients it has been necessary to actually resect breast tissue because of slow, long-term hypertrophy of the breast. These changes are related to general increases in body size, in habitus, and are associated with weight gain over a period of years.

If a patient requests simple removal and capsulectomy, this is performed through the original incision, unless it is an axillary one. If the patient requests repositioning with a new prosthesis, the circumareolar elevation may not be necessary but it is often advantageous to use the techniques of internal repair described in Chapter 10. For those patients who prefer not to have any breast prosthesis, who reject either textured gel prosthesis replacement or textured saline prosthesis replacement, the circumareolar technique is offered. We discuss this in detail with illustrations and assurances that the breast, although smaller, will retain much of the natural shape.

Technique

The majority of my patients are operated on in our clinic with ketamine-diazepam (Valium) dissociative anesthesia. Care is taken to block around the prosthesis because there are medicolegal concerns if the prosthesis is broken or intact. (In my experience, x-ray evaluation has frequently been incorrect. In several more recent patients, the diagnosis of broken prosthesis has not been supported by the surgical findings.) A field block using 20-gauge spinal needles is effected and local infiltration is placed around the areolar scar. With the breast lifted away from the prosthesis, a large amount of anesthetic is in-

jected into the soft tissue and allowed to permeate the area. It may be necessary to add small, additional amounts with the tissue elevated during the procedure, but care must be taken not to damage the capsule.

If there are irregularities in the original circumareolar or periareolar scar, these areas are excised and a generous amount of soft tissue is reflected on the lower skin flap. In preparation for the mastopexy, this flap is dissected under direct vision over the lower third of the breast so that the remaining breast wall is exposed. With a hook elevating the areola, cutting cautery is used to make a direct vertical split to the inframammary fold until the capsule is encountered. Careful cautery opens the capsule so that one may ascertain whether there is liquid silicone, a broken prosthesis, or other abnormalities. If the implant is intact, the incision is lengthened and the implant is removed. At this point it is wise to inject local anesthetic beneath the posterior capsule and around the periphery through the capsule wall itself. If the implant is broken, all of the capsule and some pericapsular tissue must be removed. Gloves are changed and the capsule is then excised under direct vision.

It is useful to grasp the capsule and slide a curved, blunt-tipped scissor with a cutting and spreading motion around the capsule left, right, and superiorly as much as possible before beginning to remove the capsule. In many cases it is impossible to remove the capsule without dividing it into quadrants. The last dissection, from the underlying muscle or rib cage, is facilitated by instilling large amounts of dilute anesthetic beneath the capsule to elevate it from the underlying tissue. Bleeding points are controlled after complete capsulectomy.

If the patient has requested a circumareolar mastopexy, the outlined circle has been deepithelialized prior to entry into the breast. If a replacement without elevation of the areola is contemplated, one next evaluates the length of the two lateral walls from the areola to what will be the new inframammary fold. It is often necessary to shorten this by excising lateral wedges. The pocket is then irrigated with povidone-iodine (Betadine) and the new prosthesis is prepared.

At the time of this writing, federal guidelines

mandate that patients having breast prosthesis replacement may choose between silicone implants filled with modern gel or silicone implants filled with saline. Because of the risk of deflation and the thicker wall of the saline prosthesis, we counsel our patients in their choices. My personal preference is for the gel-filled prosthesis.

It has become apparent in 1994 that fewer contractures occur with textured-wall prostheses than with smooth-walled ones. We now use only textured-wall prostheses even though they are often more palpable. Saline textured prostheses are overinflated by 20 to 30% to reduce the incidence of visible or palpable rippling.

Implant Rupture Detection

Rupture of a breast prosthesis is not an easy diagnosis. It has become clear that the only true diagnostic test is opening the capsule and having a look! There have been false positives and false negatives, which is not uncommon with any diagnostic procedure, but it is certainly frustrating for the breast implant patient.

For example, in one of our patients, the X-ray was diagnostic for a ruptured prosthesis: there was a "balloon" of material outside the smooth shell of the implant. Because her implants were made in 1979 and are now known to become more fragile with time, we advised implant removal. The implant was intact but one corner was in a thinner part of the breast wall (Figure 11.1).

The second difficulty is that implants may be ruptured but the silicone may be enclosed by a dense fibrous capsule. As long as the free silicone material remains within the capsule it is more of a nuisance than a problem. Once it escapes (Figure 11.2) there may be an intense soft tissue reaction. In several cases free liquid silicone has migrated along tissue paths and surfaced in the shoulder or forearm. Once it reaches a certain spot, such as the axillary crease, a foreign body reaction begins and the patient notices a palpable mass. In one of our cases, this mass appeared 3 years following her implant replacement for rupture.

The more common problem is exudation of silicone in a semiliquid form through an intact

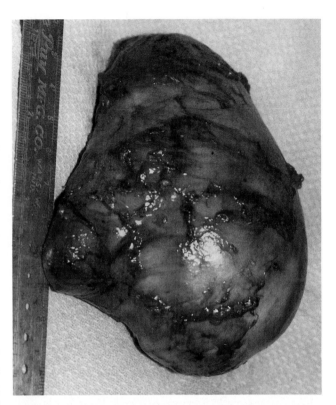

Figure 11.1. One of the problems in mammography is that the outline and thickness of the capsule are the only positive information that one may gather. In this case both the radiologist and I were certain that this patient had a ruptured prosthesis. There was the typical appearance of a tight capsule, and a "ballooning" of capsular material into the adjacent breast mass. To our surprise, we found that the implant was indeed tightly encapsulated but, as shown here, the ballooning was simply a result of bands within the breast; Cooper's suspensory ligaments may be quite well developed. With time and pressure the prosthesis may balloon between them without actually breaking, and such was the case here. Nevertheless, replacement with a textured wide-based gel restored her to the desired shape, softness, and comfort.

prothesis, with isolated siliconoma formation (Figure 11.2). In the patient illustrated in Figure 11.2 there are two small areas that show the typical foamy appearance of siliconoma, indicating a foreign body reaction. We know today that this reaction will continue and become more than just a simple diagnostic dilemma.

A general surgeon diagnosed the patient in Figure 11.3 as having a "cyst" and was prepared to aspirate it. This would have had disastrous

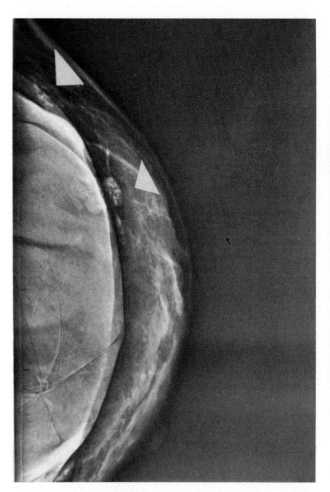

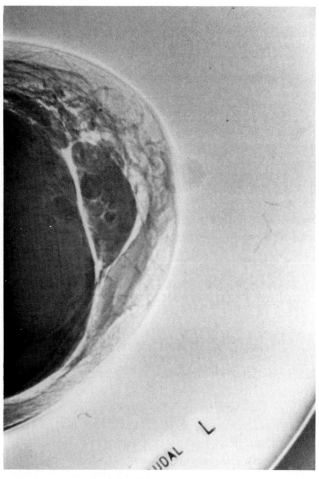

Figure 11.2. Bracketed by the arrowheads are true siliconomas. The characteristic foamy appearance indicates that a greater degree of silicone seepage has occurred, and/or the actual shell of the prosthesis has broken. Silicone foreign body reaction has extended beyond the 2-mm penetration of "silicone bleed." These small siliconomas are frequently palpable and are usually removed to eliminate the possibility of a misdiagnosis.

Figure 11.3. Silicone extruding from a prosthesis can resemble a cyst, leading to a misdiagnosis.

consequences because, as the X-ray shows, this is extruded silicone from a 1977 prosthesis. This patient had had no difficulties, no encapsulation, and no history of trauma.

Silicone extravasation through an intact implant occurs with all silicone prostheses but to a minor and only microscopically detectable degree. Some of the early prostheses manufactured between 1962 and 1975 "sweated" a significant amount of silicone, which elicited a calcific capsular reaction (Figure 11.4). Breast augmentation

patients in the first 15 years were expected to have firm, hard breasts. X-ray examination lagged behind with the development of xerograms and current imaging and enlarging techniques, and the use of the Ekland maneuver, in which the breast is lifted away from the chest wall for better imaging, and radiologists are more comfortable with breast prostheses. Admittedly, it is more difficult for them when the breast is calcified or encapsulated to a degree causing painfulness (Figure 11.5).

Figure 11.4. This X-ray shows a typical appearance of excess silicone bleed, to which the breast has responded with fibrosis and ultimate calcification. Although this calcification is not indicative of further problems that would develop, it does compromise mammography. Silicone bleed of this degree is not seen with modern prostheses. It indicates that the liquid element of the gel material penetrated no more than 1 or 2 mm beyond the forming capsule.

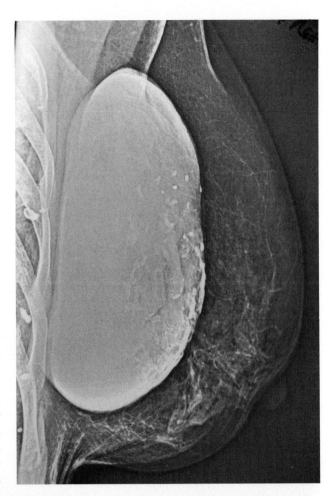

Figure 11.5. *Left:* A normal prosthesis dating from 1974. *Right:* A characteristic finding of a ruptured prosthesis with intense foreign body reaction. The convolutions in the shape of the prosthesis are indicative of rupture and do not require magnetic resonance imaging analysis to confirm the diagnosis. A second diagnostic factor is illustrated here: the image on X-ray is much larger than the original diameter of the 1974 prostheses. In these cases, an extensive subcutaneous removal of soft tissue is required, often with complex rotation flaps or even submuscular placement to restore the breast and prevent further migration of the silicone. In my experience, this intense foreign body reaction usually occurs within 1 year. This is based on several cases in which definite trauma elicited an appearance that was diagnosed but surgery was declined by the patient until the emergence of a foreign body reaction.

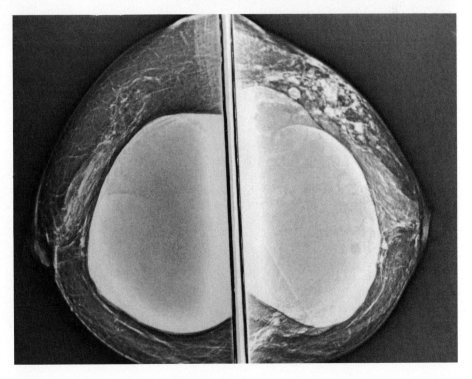

Prosthesis Removal With Circumareolar Mastopexy

Although some patients have requested implant removal in response to media misinformation about the dangers of breast prostheses, many patients have requested implant removal for other, more logical reasons. Patient J.S. is shown in 1992 (Figure 11.6A–C), some 10 years following breast augmentation. Hers was a type C-1 breast augmentation (see Chapter 1 for a discussion of categories), in which a ptotic breast is enlarged as a measure to achieve normalcy without mastopexy. One year later, however, she began to notice more weight-related symptoms and, with her concern about breast implant safety, requested implant removal. There had been some noticeable increase in size and only moderate descent (Figure 11.6D–F). In patients with thicker breasts, a reasonably full contour may be obtained by the infolding technique after removal of the prosthesis and its capsule. The result is an acceptable breast (Figure 11.6G and H) with smaller areolae and uplifted shape.

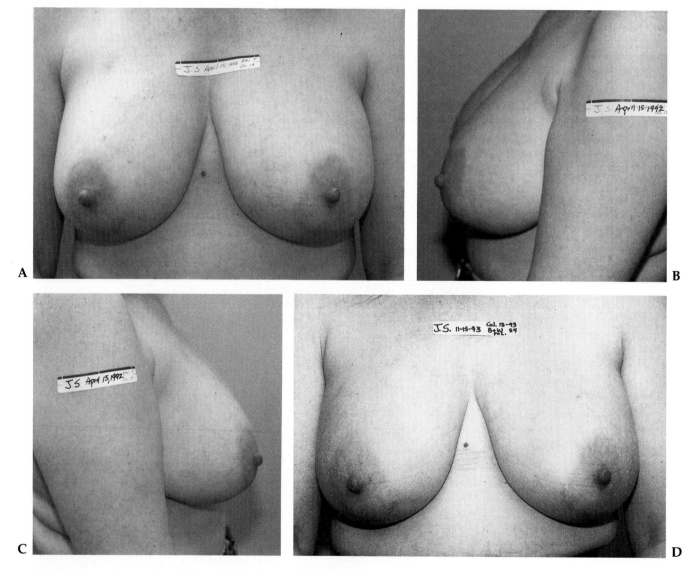

Figure 11.6. Breast implant removal. See text for details.

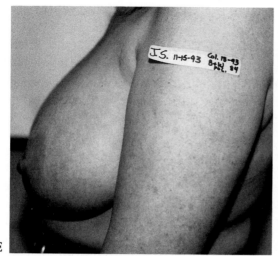

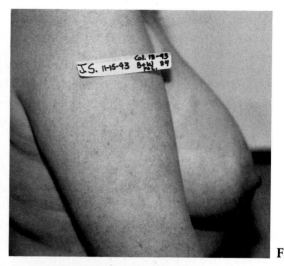

E

F

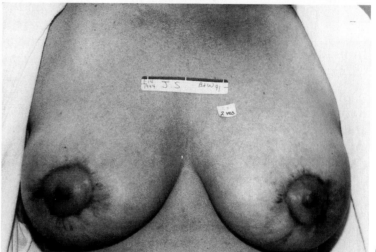

G

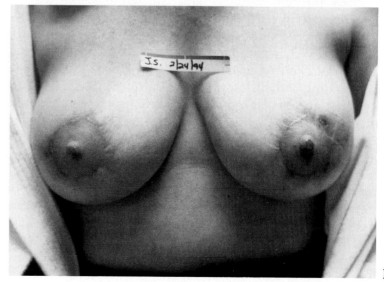

H

Patients who have implants removed are already frightened and angry and it is not in their best interest to leave more visible scarring with the standard inverted T mastopexy maneuvers. Even those whose removals will result in breasts much smaller than those of this patient should be spared the unnecessary problem of dealing with more exposed scars on the chest wall.

In the patients shown in Figures 11.7 and 11.8, the internal mound exposes the previously hidden area beneath the original breast ptosis; a T scar would be visible, and more annoying as a reminder to these patients of the loss they have suffered. The delayed smoothing of the circle is a small price to pay.

Implant Replacement With Circumareolar Mastopexy

If the areola needs to be repositioned and shortening of the stretched skin laterally and medially needs to be effected, the deepithelialized circle technique is performed prior to entry into the capsule. Left-to-right reinforcement is used as noted in Chapter 10, but it is often necessary to separate skin from the edge of the deepithelialized circle after this maneuver is completed. This is effected around the periphery even to the two o'clock position medially and the ten o'clock position laterally. This depends on the size of the circle. At this point, the double Benelli sutures are employed, beginning with the nonabsorbable suture placed at a distance from the skin edges and ending with the absorbable 2-0 suture placed in the subcuticular position. Drains are rarely necessary.

In response to a survey for the journal that I edit, *Technical Forum* (Journal of the International Society of Clinical Plastic Surgeons, 1993), we received several replies from readers who were certain that the mammography process itself had broken an old and fragile prosthesis.

The use of magnetic resonance imaging is no longer controversial. Although there are false positives and false negatives, this technique is limited only by the cost of the procedure. In my practice, it is advised only if a patient has an absolutely soft prosthesis that we suspect is broken, and prefers not to have an exploration and replacement.

Several features of the physical examination may indicate that a breast prosthesis is changed. The most reliable is a patient's own evaluation of changes in her breasts. A sudden onset of pain, surface reddening, or a change in shape or consistency may be suggestive; a history of trauma is not necessary to make a diagnosis of probable implant rupture. This rule applies to implants manufactured between 1970 and 1984. The implants of the 1960s were so firm that they could not rupture except under extreme stress. Implants manufactured from 1985 to the present are made with a thicker capsule and a more cohesive material. We have seen several patients in 1993 who have suffered broken ribs from automobile trauma. The implants did not break and perhaps saved them from further injury.

The second physical examination test that may be useful is a figure trapping maneuver. If fingers are pressed against the chest wall and the implant is moved upward, an intact implant will not pass beyond the fingers. A broken implant with free silicone will, of course, move between the fingers. I have found this test useful.

It must also be stated that there are individuals whose X-rays show migration of silicone into the axilla, but who have absolutely no foreign body reaction. In these cases, the material that we remove has the consistency of motor oil and there is surprisingly little reaction. Other patients, who have been in automobile accidents and for whom the diagnosis of broken implant was made, resisted the advice for replacement and later developed multiple siliconomas. Although this is not dangerous physically, it is certainly more difficult for the surgeon to remove this tissue and reconstruct the breast.

In summary, then, if an adequate radiological examination shows signs that suggest implant rupture, and the implant was manufactured between 1970 and 1984, surgical exploration is indicated. The patient may then choose a new prosthesis of the silicone saline or silicone gel type, or may opt for simple removal. Other patients, particularly those who have slowly enlarged, thickened breast tissue, may choose to have a

Figures 11.7 and 11.8. Patients from whom implants were removed without additional residual scarring.

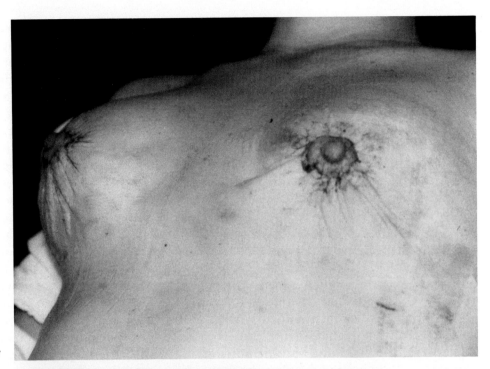

Figure 11.7

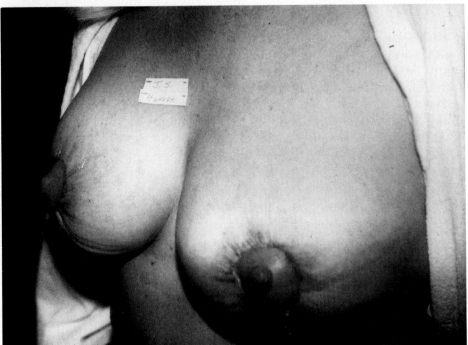

Figure 11.8

circumareolar mastopexy after implant removal. The same choices apply to patients in whom the X-ray examination does not provide sufficient information for a diagnosis of ruptured prosthesis, but who nonetheless present physical evidence of prosthetic rupture. In one recent case the diagnosis was made only by the observation that her 1976 prosthesis was not as large vertically or horizontally as the X-ray image. This indicated that the capsule had broken and that the implant material was free. In another recent case, the X-ray diagnosis was unequivocable and even though we found cohesive gel, there were areas of intense siliconoma formation. This patient chose to undergo revision of her old mastopexy augmentation and added a 350-cm^3 textured gel prosthesis to fit her lifestyle and self-image.

I recommend that each patient who is counseled regarding implant integrity should receive copies of all pertinent medical literature so that she may be fully informed before she makes her decision. Then, if she chooses implant removal, I will discuss the choices of circumareolar mastopexy, simple removal, or removal and replacement. According to Food and Drug Administration (FDA) guidelines, there is no reason to remove a breast prosthesis unless it is ruptured, and patients who are undergoing replacement or repair may choose between saline-filled or gel-filled prostheses. Reports[7–9] in the plastic surgery literature between 1991 and 1994 indicate that these patients, who traditionally have a higher incidence of capsular contracture following replacements, actually experience a much lower incidence of contracture if textured prostheses are used. Patients must be counseled about the differences between "modern" and original prostheses. The advantages of the saline prosthesis are that it can be adjusted in surgery and can be inserted through a much smaller incision. The disadvantage is that the smooth-walled saline prostheses are associated with a greater capsular contracture rate than the textured wall prostheses, but both are palpable and occasionally visible. This rippling usually occurs in the lower quadrants, an area that cannot be covered by submuscular placement. My practice is to avoid submuscular placement whenever possible and to use overfilling as a partial remedy.

The gel-filled textured prostheses are rarely visible, even though rippling can be detected by palpation. They do not have the parchment-like feel under the skin and, of course, there is no danger of deflation. Patients who choose saline prosthetic replacement must be made aware that current reports indicate a spontaneous deflation rate of between 2 and 10%.

Once my patient has read all of the literature that we have prepared regarding research on silicones, as well as epidemiological surveys and studies on the incidence of malignancy, and have actually seen and held textured prostheses of both types, the choice can be made. A few of these patients wish to have additional incisions. Most of them have invisible scars in the periareolar zone and many have assured me that their husbands do not know that they have had surgery. If the prosthesis is intact and there is no evidence on physical examination or X-ray, they are advised of an additional choice: leave the prosthesis alone and reevaluate it on a yearly basis. Many have chosen this option.

Those that choose replacement often require repositioning of the areola or a full circumareolar mastopexy. Others simply require a wider prosthesis and removal of any capsular contracture that may be present. A small number will have an acceptable shape if the prosthesis is removed, owing to later thickening and enlargement of the breast. I believe it is unconscionable not to use the original scar. These patients are under emotional stress and the addition of a second scar for the convenience of the surgeon cannot be defended. With experience, complete capsulectomy, with or without replacement, is not a difficult procedure through the original or a new, short periareolar procedure.

Whether or not to do a complete capsulectomy depends on the appearance of the capsule. If a patient has an older gel-type prosthesis with capsule thickening and/or calcification, a complete capsulectomy is required. I try to leave capsular tissue laterally, to reinforce against lateral drift into the anterior axillary lines. There is usually an abundance of good tissue inferiorly, so that the capsule may be resected in all other areas and particularly superiorly. Injecting dilute lidocaine (Xylocaine) beneath the posterior capsule allows easy removal from the muscle without tearing or bleeding.

Today, we replace the implant with a textured-type prosthesis because it tends to hold its position for a longer period of time. Implants are chosen on the basis of the width of the patient's chest and the patient's desire for fullness and cleavage.

In January 1980 I wrote a short editorial in *Technical Forum* entitled, "And They Told Us There Were No 'Liquid' Silicone Radicals in the Gel."[10] Many of us were surprised to find intact breast prostheses covered by 10 to 20 cc of extremely sticky liquid silicone. We began to see patients with enlarged axillary lymph nodes and occasional small siliconomas that I described at that point as "embolic" lumps of semiliquid silicone. This is not a problem for surgeons today. The current breast prostheses are of either the saline-filled type or the gel-filled type, which do not have the problem of transmigration of liquid silicone or frequent rupture.

Simple Replacement With Internal Repair

The capsular space is fully expanded superiorly and laterally. Sharp dissection is used only superiorly and blunt dissection is used laterally and medially to preserve nerve supply. Additional expansion of this tissue is easily effected when the prosthesis is in place. Pressure with a retractor in all quadrants further expands the breast tissue to allow the prosthesis of choice to fit easily into the new space. The limbs of the left and right breast wall have been shortened to 6 cm. With the prosthesis in position, the leading edge of the lateral wall is sutured to the underlying muscle at the new position and two tacking stitches are placed along the horizontal line. The remaining portion of the wall is sutured to the undersurface of the medial section, which is now overlapped and sutured into place, giving double protection and double reinforcement of the new inframammary fold. Minor loosening of skin attachment subcutaneously is often required so that the skin of the breast will fall into position when it is being resutured. A small catheter is placed into the pocket for later installation of bupivacaine hydrochloride (Marcaine), methylprednizolone (Solu-Medrol), and cephalothin (Keflin). The use of antibiotics and steroids, although perhaps ineffective, has seemed to reduce complications. We know that bacteria have been liberated by the incision through the breast parenchyma and that our povidone-iodine (Betadine) irrigation will stay in the tissues for several weeks, but the addition of an antibiotic solution is certainly reassuring to the surgeon. The incidences of infection in modern surgery remain quite low, although one in all honesty may ascribe this to improvements in techniques and materials rather than to suffusion of tissue with antibiotics during surgery, followed by oral administration of antibiotics.

The edge of the areola is then backcut a few millimeters so that it will be everted when the skin is repositioned. A deep layer of inverted Dexon 4-0 sutures brings a soft tissue shelf into contact with the shelf of soft tissue beneath the areolar edge. A second horizontal layer of Dexon 4-0 sutures brings this tissue together and a final layer of subcuticular Dexon 5-0 sutures is used to further evert the edges and reduce all tension.

Implant Removal With Internal Mastopexy

Fortunately, most patients who wish to have their implants removed completely will either accept a smaller breast or have such hypertrophy of the soft tissue that a good cone may be created with the Erol infolding technique. The procedure begins with the deepithelialization of the circle, followed by separation of the soft tissue so that the remaining wall of the breast is exposed.

After capsulectomy and removal of the prosthesis through the vertical splitting incision, it is often advantageous to fold under the additional soft tissue rather than resect it. This is the soft tissue that makes up the excessive length between the areola and the new inframammary fold. As in "bending the knee," the edge of this soft tissue is brought upward and sutured in its highest possible position so that the remaining 5 to 6 cm still fits at the position of the new infra-

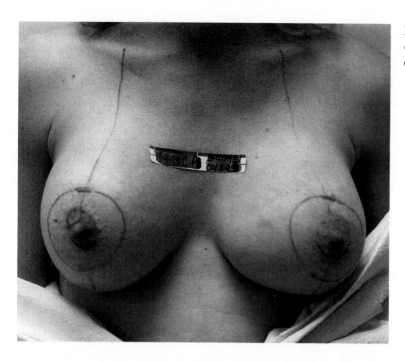

Figure 11.9. The amount of skin removed during implant removal is less than during circumareolar mastopexy.

mammary fold. At the same time, the split edges are infolded on themselves as much as possible. There are several methods by which to infold this tissue; the object of all of them is to move as much of the breast wall into a position directly beneath the areola as possible. The bending and infolding techniques, both inferiorly and medially, have worked best for me. In certain cases we have so much soft tissue that it is easy to resect a portion inferiorly and still infold the entire breast tissue to create a C cup. Once the external sutures have been placed, creating the subcutaneous cone, the skin closure is performed as described above.

As illustrated in Figure 11.9, patients undergoing implant removal do not require a great deal of skin removal, and therefore the circle can be much smaller. Because the breast prosthesis has been in place for years, there is not the same concern for blood supply as in a circumareolar mastopexy with the addition of a prosthesis. In those cases, one must be certain not to interrupt blood supply because the main portion of the breast is being undermined for the prosthesis and the skin and subcutaneous tissue of the lower half have been separated. In the replacement patient, the blood supply is secure.

Note that the areola will be elevated a short distance. Because there is less tissue to create the new mound, only the deepithelialized dermis is removed in the triangle above the areola. As opposed to circumareolar mastopexy with augmentation, it is unnecessary to remove a deeper triangular wedge of tissue to avoid the dome shape that was characteristic of the early cases.

Internal Repair and Standard Mastopexy Revision Following Implant Removal

Patient C.F. (Figure 11.10) underwent a mastopexy in 1984 with breast prostheses and almost immediately began to experience tightening on the right side. As was often the case in the mid-1980s, fibrosis continued and despite several revisions and the use of a double-lumen prosthesis the capsular contracture recurred (Figure 11.10A–C).

Our practice in the mid-1980s was to use polyurethane prostheses for recalcitrant fibrous capsular contracture, and this was our choice of treatment in 1987 for patient C.F. The left side had never tightened but had slowly descended. Unfortunately, the capsular contracture on the right returned with a vengeance shortly after the Replicon (Surgitech-Medical Engineering Corp.,

Figure 11.10. See text for details.

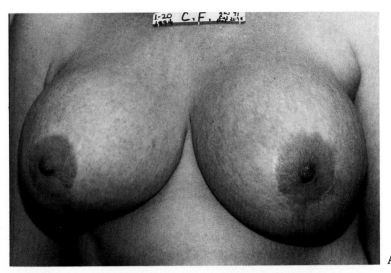

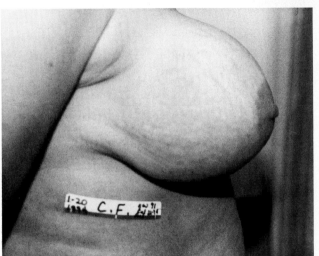

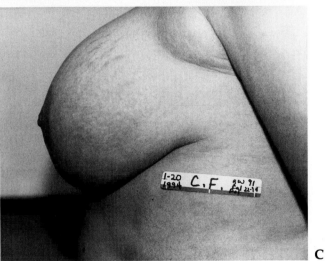

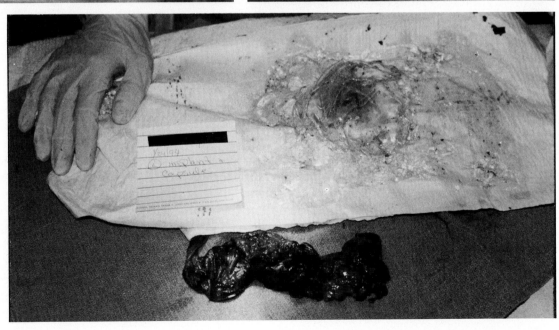

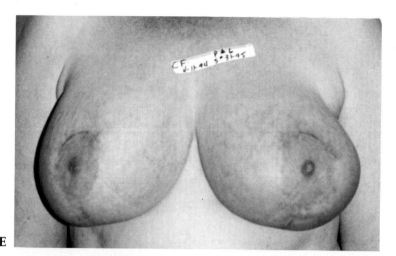

Figure 11.10. *Continued*

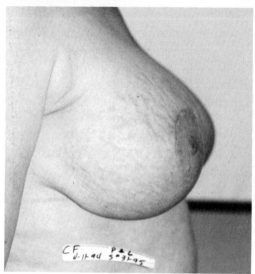

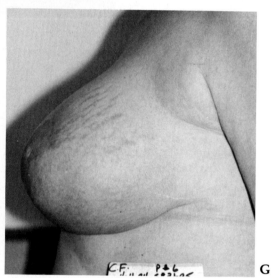

Racine, WI) polyurethane-covered prostheses were placed in 1987.

Despite the fact that the right breast had had five surgeries and the left retained the original 1984 255-cm³ gel prosthesis, we made another attempt to restore her that was completely successful. As shown in Figure 11.10A–C, the patient had presented asymmetry with retraction on the right side and descent on the left. There was a discrepancy in nipple position. A crescent lift was performed on the right side with a complete internal release of all scar tissue and a capsulectomy, removing all of the polyurethane prosthetic capsule (Figure 11.10D). A 350-cm³ textured gel row-bleed prosthesis was positioned on the right side in the correct inframammary

fold spot. When the crescent was closed the nipple-areolar complex was brought up to a position that would be matched by a revision of the left side. The left-side prosthesis was found to be ruptured, with adjacent siliconoma formation (Figure 11.10D).

When scars are present from a standard mastopexy, it is wise to proceed with standard mastopexy revision, which includes removal of the scar and a deep layer left-to-right closure after skin excision. To reset the areola, we simply deepithelialized the circle and moved the areola into position, thus preserving greater blood supply and fullness in the flattened supraareolar position. A 350-cm³ textured gel prothesis was then positioned on the left at a higher spot (Fig-

Figure 11.11. Genuflexion procedure. See text for details.

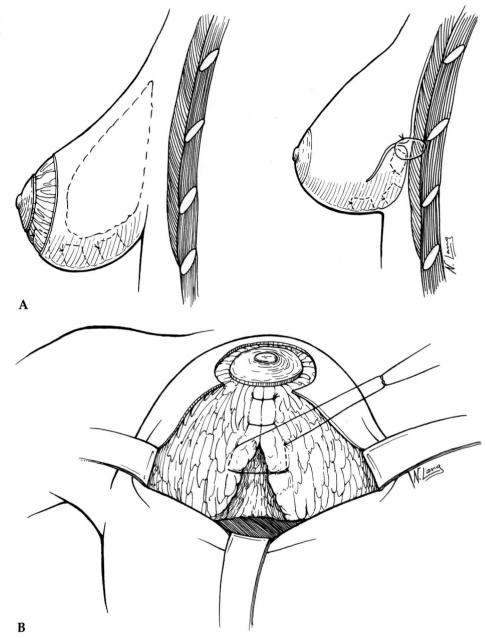

A

B

ure 11.10E–G) than the original because the inframammary fold had now been reset. Figure 11.10E–F shows the relative symmetry that has been obtained.

In this patient a circumareolar adjustment was not required because the nipple shape was essentially normal and the stretching had occurred from the nipple to the inframammary fold on the left side. The use of a textured prosthesis gave the advantage of anchoring the new breast prosthe-

ses at comparable positions on the left and right sides. There has been no occurrence of capsular contracture and breast softness and symmetry are greatly improved.

Genuflection Procedure

When a patient requests prosthesis removal after a period of years, there is usually excess tissue owing to gravitational stretch. The distance between the new areolar site and the new inframmary fold may measure as much as 10 cm. The excess tissue is rotated beneath the central core of the breast to aid in formation of a projecting mound.

As shown in Figure 11.11A, the first step is to deepithelialize a small circle so that the areola may be repositioned. With the skin reflected one can easily ascertain the correct point for placement of the infolding suture. I begin by splitting the breast vertically, so that the capsule and prosthesis can be removed. The point is fixed and marked at 6 cm and this portion of the breast wall will be fixed to the point designating the new inframammary fold. The first suture, as shown, infolds the soft tissue beneath the breast as in flexing of the knee (genuflection).

With this tissue firmly secured in a high position the additional infolding sutures may be placed as described elsewhere in text (see Chapter 7). Following placement of the infolding sutures in one or two layers, as shown in Figure 11.11B, a series of sutures is placed to secure the breast at the new inframammary fold in its uplifted position.

Figure 11.11A shows an alternative that may be useful. The vertical split is repaired first, to gauge the amount of tissue that is present in case one wishes to trim away some of the "genuflect" infolding to reduce the volume of the breast. In the majority of cases I prefer to make the genuflection fixation before closing and infolding anteriorly.

✤ 12 ✤

Problems and Problem Solving

Tolbert S. Wilkinson

Introduction

If the only problems with the circumareolar reduction/mastopexy/repair surgeries were the occasional stitch granuloma, as illustrated in Figure 12.1, there would be no question that the procedure is vastly superior to standard surgeries. As readers know, patients gain and lose weight, the breast stretches or contracts, fibrocystic disease interferes with prostheses, and scars often behave erratically. The same psychological problems are seen. Patients whose breasts are reduced often have a change of heart and ask for further enlargement. Those who have implants removed are sometimes no longer content with the breast size that is achieved by utilizing all of their remaining breast tissue. These problems are independent of the surgical procedure and are not always avoided by extensive preoperative counseling. The problem of capsular contracture has become less of a concern with the advent of textured prostheses and improvement in control of bacterial overgrowth.

In addition to cases such as those illustrated in this chapter, the surgeon performing circumare-

olar mastopexies will still encounter asymmetries of the areola, just as occur occasionally with standard mastopexy and reduction, and irregularities of scarring. The percentage of patients who require revisions of areolar shape or scar hypertrophy seems to be less today than in the past, and certainly is encountered less often than with standard T scar surgeries.

Case I: Stitch Granuloma and Spot Purulence

In addition to stitch granuloma, the patient shown in Figure 12.1 also has one of the minor complications of the circumareolar technique: small purulent spots at the folds. In this case, only the left side was involved. As shown here (5 weeks after surgery), these areas are a nuisance and are often multifocal when they occur. Simply cleansing, followed by topical applications of drying agents such as merbromin leads to quick resolution. Because the suture closest to this area is absorbable, the process of "spitting" is not a concern. Surprisingly, patients who have suf-

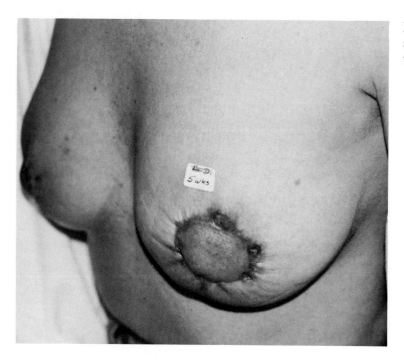

Figure 12.1. Case I: Stitch subsequent to circumareolar reduction mastopexy.

fered this complication go on to form acceptable scars that are indistinguishable from those on the opposite side.

Case II: Secondary Circumareolar Reduction for Continued Asymmetry

Patient M.A.F. underwent a breast augmentation on the hypoplastic right side and a circumareolar infolding Erol-type mastopexy on the left in 1984 (Figure 12.2A). Symmetry was achieved for many years, but by 1991 the left breast had continued to enlarge and the right had enlarged also (Figure 12.2B). This change in texture and content now gave her symptoms of breast weight, with neck and back pain. In her 1991 evaluation, it was decided to further reduce the left side by subcutaneous Pitanguy wedge excision and resetting of the gland, and to remove the prosthesis on the right side completely. We would then reconstruct the right side with whatever tissue was available,

and reduce the left side to match. She was fully aware that this would result in a much smaller size than could be achieved by the addition of a small prosthesis on the right.

Figure 12.2C and D shows the areas for deepithelialization on the left and right sides, and the areas for liposuction within the breasts and in the axillary folds. After completing the infolding of all existing tissue on the right side and the preliminary wedge resection and circumareolar reduction on the left, the left side was still visibly larger, as shown in Figure 12.2E. A 4-mm Cobra-type liposuction cannula was then introduced through the drain site and suction was performed to bring the breast down to the size shown in Figure 12.2F and G. Tape support was discontinued at the end of $2\frac{1}{2}$ weeks, but brassiere support was maintained continuously for the following month. The final results (see Figure 12.2H, patient shown in her brassiere) have been maintained. At 6 months, the last edema from the liposuction was resolving nicely and the symmetry is now quite acceptable.

Figure 12.2. Case II: Secondary circumareolar reduction for continued asymmetry. See text for details.

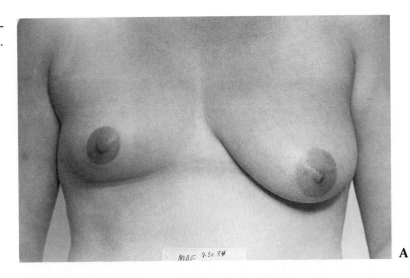

A

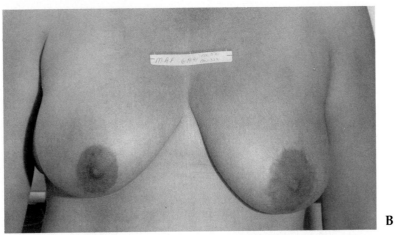

B

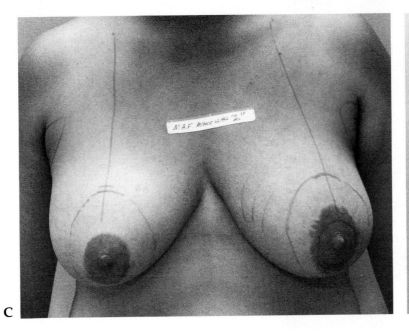

C

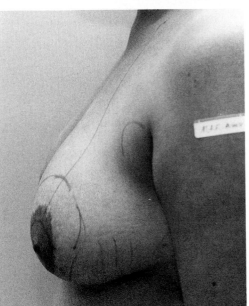

D

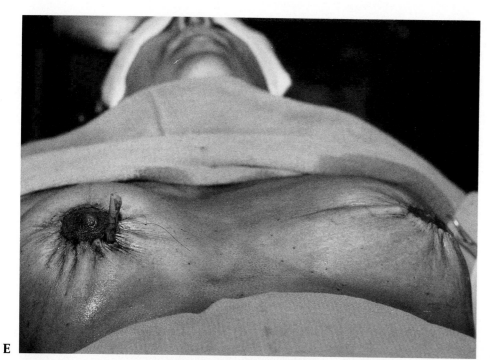

Figure 12.2. *Continued*

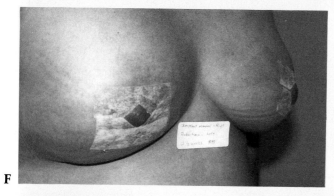

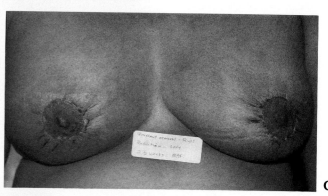

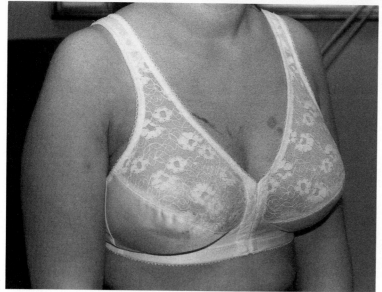

Case III: Internal Repair and Pregnancy

Patient A.J. (Figure 12.3A–C) is a professional nudist with ptotic breasts. Our initial discussion in 1986 concerned the effect of lack of brassiere support on the breast type that we call type C (see Chapter 1 for a more detailed discussion of breast typing). Our breast augmentation patients are divided into type A (very flat, very fibrotic), type B (the most common, with moderate stretchability and minor ptosis), and type C, as illustrated by this patient. Type C ptotic patients are offered the choice of simple augmentation with lowering of the inframammary fold, crescent mastopexy, or, in the extreme case, circumareolar mastopexy. This patient chose the first because of her activities and because her profession required that she appear topless in public. All went well and initial reports were very gratifying.

Two years later I received an anguished phone call indicating that the patient had been rejected for a photographic shoot because of extreme ptosis. Of course, she admitted that she had not worn a brassiere since the day she left Texas to return to her native state. I advised her to return as quickly as possible so that we could do a repositioning with the internal repair procedure discussed in this book. As expected, we found that the lower portions of her breasts had stretched the most, while the areolar position had changed by only a few centimeters (Figure 12.3D–F). She asked if a photographer would be able to see her incisions and my reply was, "Did he see the original ones?" With her enthusiastic reply in the negative, we were able to proceed with the internal support and a wider, fuller prosthesis to take up some of the discrepancy. I saw the patient again in her home state (with my long-suffering wife in attendance), during an Educational Foundation Symposium at which I served as a faculty member. I was able to ascertain that there had been no further descent and that her breasts were as natural in appearance as the photographic shoot had shown them to be 2 years earlier. This, it would seem, was a happy ending to the story. She was again cautioned about brassiere support.

Unfortunately, not all stories have such happy endings. In January 1994 she again returned to my clinic with the request, "Can you do something?" She had changed her profession to topless dancer and had had her first pregnancy, both of which are known to accelerate ptosis of the breast. As shown in Figure 12.3G and H, her breast tissue had continued to descend. The choices at this point were quite limited.

When this degree of descent has occurred certain patients may choose enlargement to a D-cup breast size because it suits their particular needs at that time, even though it is not the aesthetic result that I would highly recommend. She was adamant that this was her view as well. This left only one choice: circumareolar mastopexy with repositioning of the inframammary fold, shortening of the areola-to-mammary fold distance, and elevation and reduction of the areola. She wanted to continue with her lucrative career but, to my surprise, turned down the proposed surgery for a reason that I had not suspected. In her home state, "entertainers" are not allowed to wear pasties. These small, adhesive round patches are used in Texas to cover the nipple-areolar complex and would have hidden the scar during the period of maturation. In her state and in her profession, circumareolar mastopexy would have ended her career!

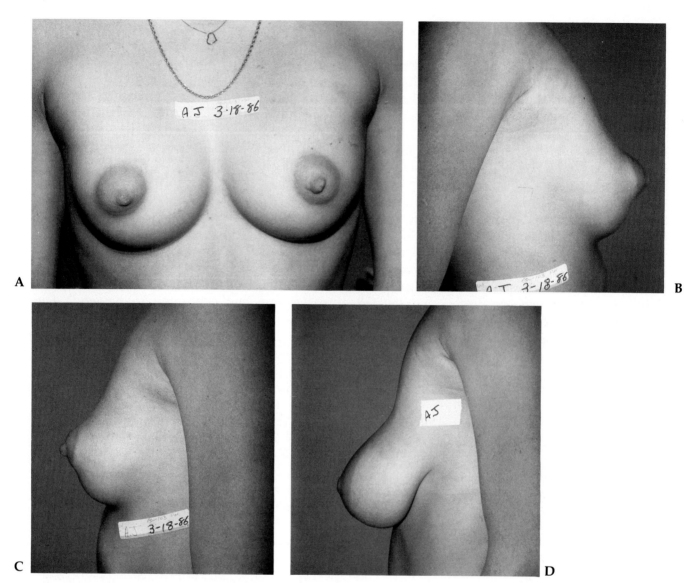

Figure 12.3. Case III: Internal repair of ptosis exacerbated by pregnancy and reluctance to wear brassieres. See text for details.

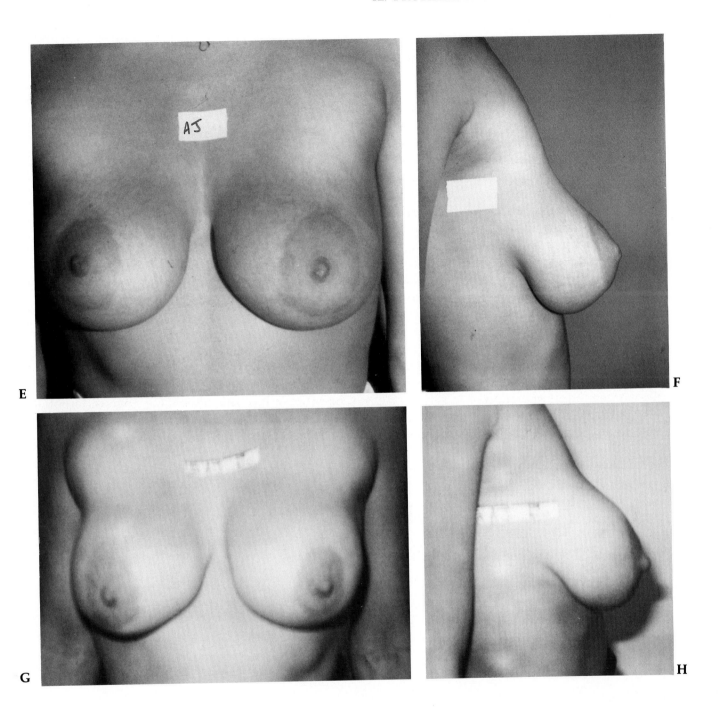

E

F

G

H

Case IV: Scar Retraction and Asymmetry in a Young Breast Reduction Patient

Younger patients are often the most vehement in opposing the use of horizontal or vertical breast incisions. In this particular case (Figure 12.4), a standard reduction would have been less problematic than the circumareolar, simply because of the bizarre asymmetry and the presence of stretch marks, which indicate problems with skin contouring (Figure 12.4A). This young patient underwent a circumareolar breast reduction in June 1990 and had an uneventful recovery. Only a single circumareolar suture of the resorbable type was used. Today we use a double Benelli suture, placing the nonabsorbable suture at a distance from the skin edges to reduce the effect of skin retraction. The patient was counseled extensively regarding the size of the reduction and, on the basis of her original appearance, chose only modest reduction.

At 18 months, the breast shape was relatively close to our original plans, although the right breast appeared to be larger. At this point we would have suggested a simple liposuction, perhaps under local anesthesia, except for the fact that the areola had expanded to an unacceptable size (Figure 12.4B and C). A secondary reduction in these patients is quite easy to accomplish. A small wedge removal and liposuction on the right side with simple infolding was done. The skin of the lower halves of her breasts was undermined and advanced over the deepithelialized zone. We also chose to reduce the diameter of the new nipple, making it smaller than the 4.2 mm I had created in 1990.

A number of young patients may also surprise the surgeon by requesting a further reduction in size. On the other hand, I have often received requests for enlargement in patients who had previously been extremely displeased by the large size of their breasts! Enlargement is the easier procedure, involving the use of a breast prosthesis. In these cases the saline "textured" prosthesis has the advantage that differential expansion may be effected for a better balancing of the final appearance (Figure 12.4D).

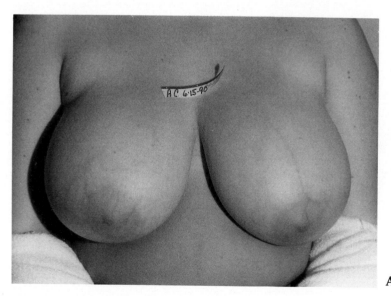

A

Figure 12.4. Case IV: Scar retraction and asymmetry in a younger patient. See text for details.

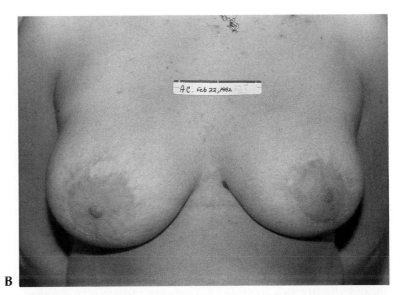

B

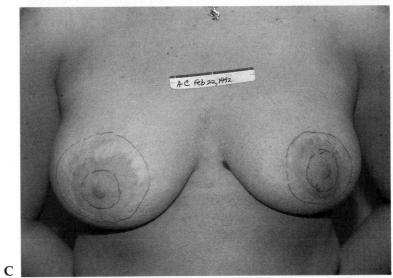

C

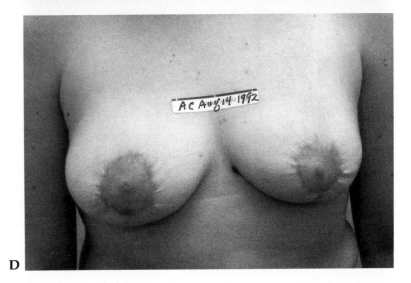

D

Case V: Continued Weight Loss Following Reduction Mammoplasty

The patient shown in Figure 12.5A and B underwent a circumareolar breast reduction to a volume that suited her, changing from a DD cup to a C cup. In 1993, 3 years later, she had lost 20 lb, with a subsequent decrease in volume of her breasts. In addition, the areolae had stretched, particularly on the left side. Her original surgery in 1990 employed only a single circumareolar suture. Note that the areolae had increased to a size larger than the original (Figure 12.5C and D).

After much discussion, we decided to retain all of the breast tissue that was still present rather than reducing her further. An areolar reduction was planned, as well as an infolding of the tissue subjacent to the areola (Figure 12.5E). This was accomplished with ketamine-diazepan (Valium) and local anesthesia.

The patient is pictured in Figure 12.5F 1 month postsurgery, with only a moderate amount of infolding still visible. The ring deepithelialization was confined to the original scar and the areolae were reduced to 3.6 mm. When the skin was reflected, an Erol-type infolding was carried out after the areolae had been moved to the more superior position at the top of the circle. This gave further projection to the breasts.

Should this patient regain the lost weight, the breasts will likely regain fullness as well. This case illustrates some of the hazards of all types of breast reductions in young adults, and the value of the double-reinforcing Benelli suture in preventing areolar expansion such as occurred here.

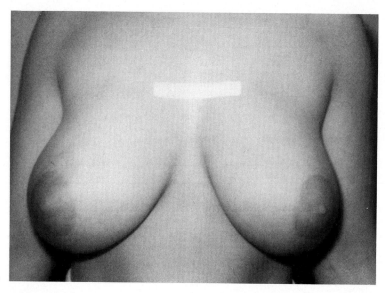
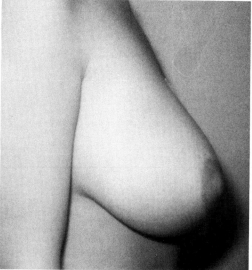

A   B

Figure 12.5. Case V: Effect of weight loss on reduction mammaplasty. See text for details.

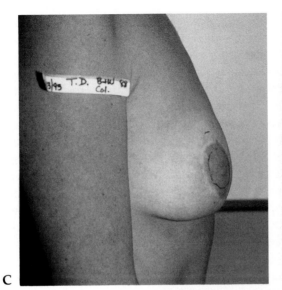

C

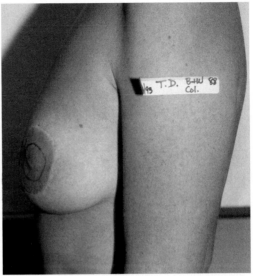

D

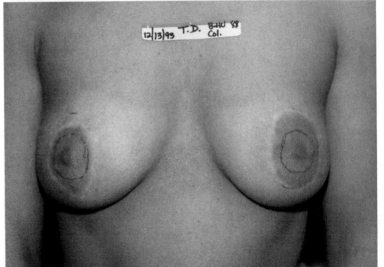

E

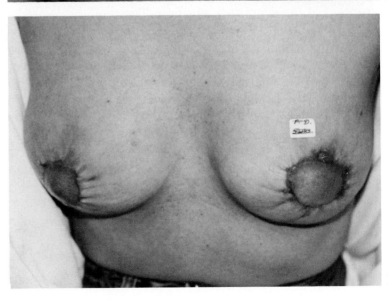

F

Case VI: The Snoopy Deformity

While looking through some old slides I found some of a patient with the classic "Snoopy" deformity. John Williams had proposed excising a circle of skin and inverting the nipple underneath, or actually infolding it on itself, to reduce the upper areola when one augmented these patients. Other authors had shown external incisions of various sorts. In this patient, I had simply expanded the undersurface of the breast with my finger tip and used a fairly good-sized implant. In the long-term photographs, the Snoopy deformity had smoothed out and the breast was conical.

I responded to an article in the *Annals of Plastic Surgery*[1] that described an external rotation flap for the Snoopy deformity. In my response I indicated that we had a long series of patients, dating back to 1972, in which an internal flap plus the presence of a breast prosthesis had given a normal rounding of the breast without the necessity of any incision except the short periareolar one. The patient that I described[2] was operated on in 1973 and still retained her original shape in 1993; in fact, her appearance is more natural than in the photographs we published! The slow descent of the breast prosthesis has accomplished this.

The areolar breast, or Snoopy deformity, is a distressing developmental anomaly found in postpubescent women. The entire breast is concentrated in an egg-sized fibrotic mass just beneath the areola. There is a depression in the contour, at the six o'clock position. The remaining breast tissue is sparse and not fibrocystic. Several techniques have been proposed for reconstruction of this defect. Each includes the use of a breast prosthesis, and most add either a ring excision of the areola or a rotation flap to fill the six o'clock defect. In my series, neither has been necessary unless the areola is gigantic in size.

In the patient shown in Figure 12.6A–F, the internal flap technique was used and the pressure of the prosthesis maintained the expansion that was created surgically. This internal flap technique (Figure 12.6G) involves moving excess tissue from the subareolar zone as a superiorly based hinge flap. During the closure after breast prosthesis positioning, this hinge flap is brought across the lower half incision line to reinforce it and eliminate the depressed zone.

This technique works well in the majority of these deformities. In others, there is an absence of fibrosis and the areola has already assumed a much larger size. In these cases one can no longer limit the incision to the short, 2-cm areola edge cut that heals so well and is almost imperceptible.

When the areola expands, the lack of fibrous tissue also contributes to late descent and further distortion of the areola, as we learned to our regret in the case shown in Figure 12.6H.

Circumareolar mastopexy techniques are most useful here, but one must emphasize the need for the double-reinforcing suture to prevent areolar stretch and that surgery cannot totally prevent breast descent. As shown in Figure 12.6H, the areola had already spread to 12 cm in diameter. It would have been wiser to have made the remaining areola smaller than shown and to use a double-reinforcing suture. At the time this patient was operated on, I was so fearful of "star gazing" that the areolae were always placed at a lower position than I would use today (Figure 12.6I).

Within 1 year further descent had occurred, as had further widening of the areola. A secondary revision (Figure 12.6J and K) was required.

The final photograph (Figure 12.6K) shows the current areolar positions, which have been maintained surprisingly well for 3 years.

Had the patient agreed with my suggestion for a wider and fuller prosthesis, the result would have been more acceptable in terms of the "ideal" silhouette. The alternative is to raise the areola to an ever higher position. The patient considered both options and has decided to leave her breasts in this configuration, a size and shape that she considers normal and attractive.

This type of circumareolar reduction is performed in a manner similar to breast repair surgeries. Once the ring has been deepithelialized, the skin flap is reflected and a pocket is created for the prosthesis by way of a vertical splitting incision. Knowing that the breasts of these younger patients will stretch with time, closure is done with a left-to-right reinforcing maneuver to

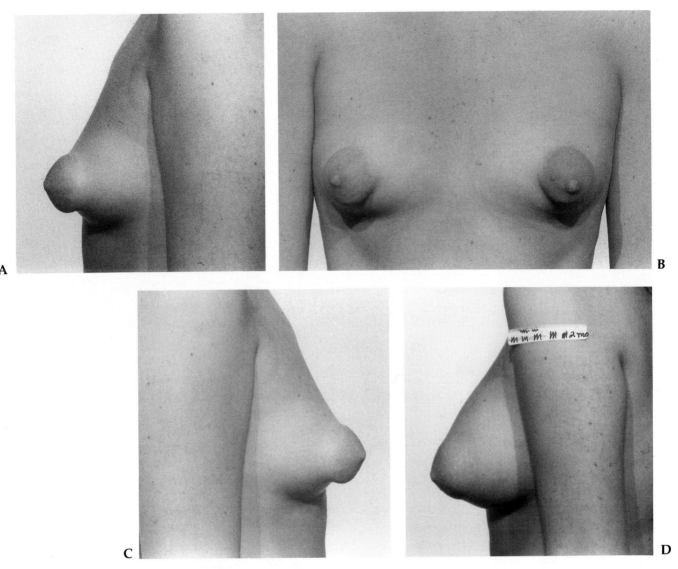

Figure 12.6. Case VI: The Snoopy deformity. See text for details.

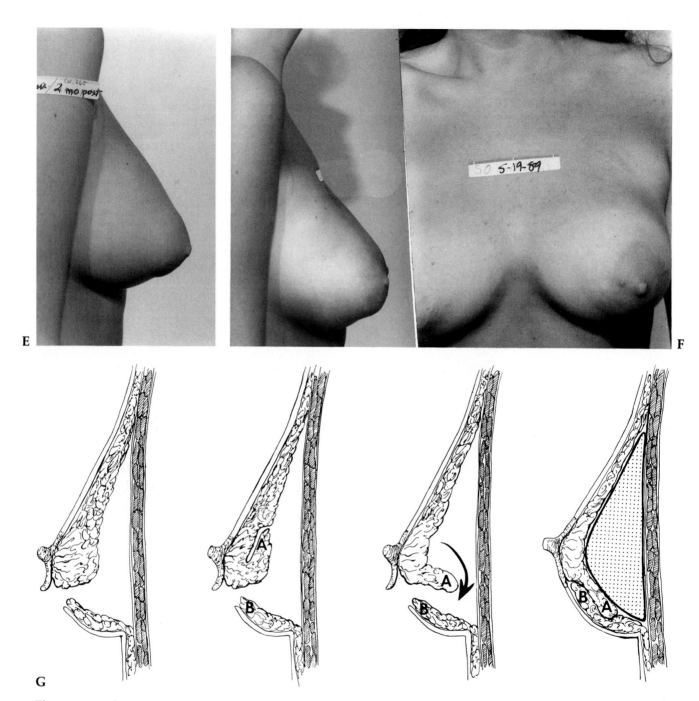

E

F

G

Figure 12.6. *Continued*

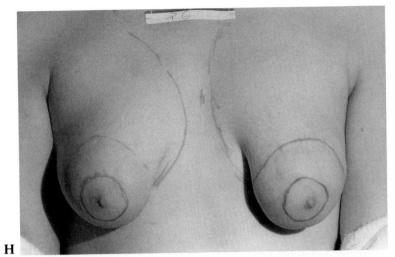

H

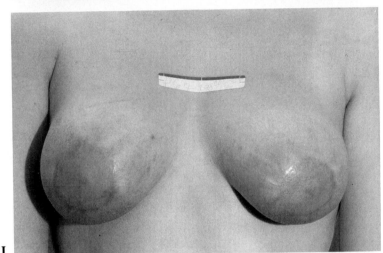

I

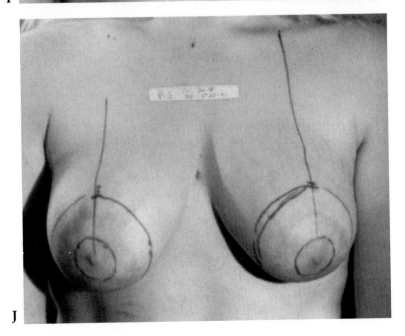

J

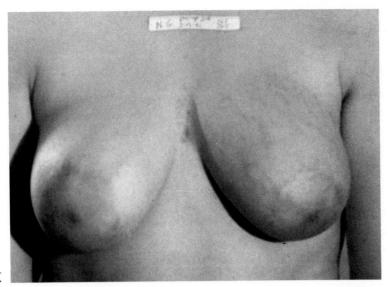

K

Figure 12.6. *Continued*

give additional thickness to the practically nonexistent lower breast wall. In my small series of patients with this deformity, descent has been inevitable but quite slow. One patient (the one with the longest follow-up), has maintained the position created by the circumareolar technique for 5 years, with no further areolar expansion and no further descent.

Case VII: Extreme Areolar Breast With Ptosis

A physician's daughter finally overcame her shyness to ask, in 1980, if something could be done about the unusual shape of her breasts (Figure 12.7A–C). The majority of her breast tissue was underneath an extremely giant areolae, and the breasts were quite ptotic. We discussed several methods of areolar reduction that she rejected. She did allow us to do a type C-2 crescent mastopexy on each side and to use a very small breast

prosthesis. Eight years later (Figure 12.7D–F) the result on the right side was reasonably acceptable but a contracture had occurred on the left, which accentuated the bizarre appearance. At this point, I felt her only alternative was a wider-based prosthesis and some form of areolar reduction.

The areolar reduction was carried out in 1988, using the single circle suture and, as was our practice then, a conservative or low areolar position was chosen.

Figure 12.7G–I shows the patient in 1993. In comparing the left lateral view, one can see that the nipple position would be better if it were more toward the upper portion of the breast, at the apex of the breast cone. This low descent was first noted in 1991. Despite discussions of aesthetics, the patient had preferred to leave the areolar position as it is shown. Surprisingly, following the original stretching of her breast in the first 8 years, there has been no further descent since the last photographs (Figure 12.7G–I) were taken.

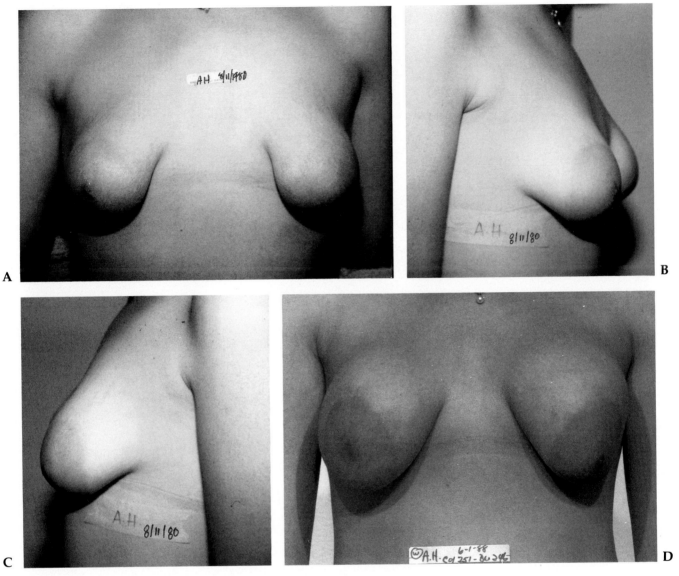

Figure 12.7. Case VII: Extreme areolar breast with ptosis. See text for details.

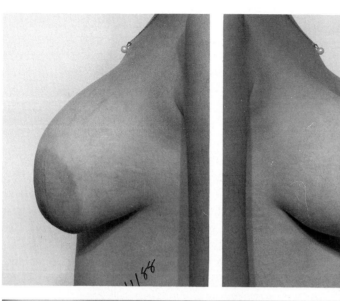

E
F

Figure 12.7. *Continued*

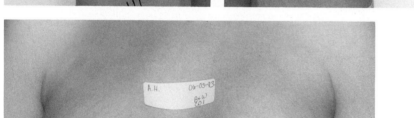

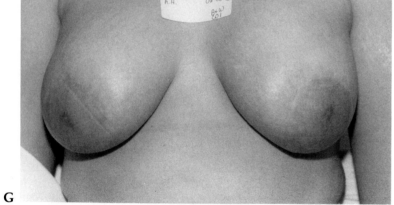

G

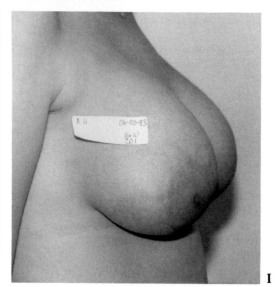

H
I

Case VIII: Bilateral Breast Augmentation and Unilateral Circumareolar Mastopexy

Patient J.H. is shown in preoperative photographs (Figure 12.8A and B) to have an unfortunately common asymmetry. The right breast is flatter than she would prefer and the left breast shows an accelerated postpartum ptosis deformity. In discussions with patients of this sort, one must emphasize that enlarging the breasts gives a greater degree of symmetry than simple unilateral mastopexy alone. Fortunately, most patients in my area (Texas) have a preconceived notion of femininity that includes medium to full C-cup breast contours. Notice the restored symmetry in the postoperative photographs (Figure 12.8C and D). On the right side a short periareolar incision has been used and a breast prosthesis added for fullness. Figure 12.6D (taken 6 months postoperatively) shows a persistence of skin folds on the left breast. These had disappeared at her last evaluation, 2 years postoperatively. The areola has been reduced to a size commensurate with the opposite side. The only difficulty was in choosing a breast prosthesis that will give a close match. In this type of mastopexy, a left-to-right cross-over closure is preferred to an infolding. I compensate by choosing a prosthesis only slightly smaller than that of the right side. The additional bulk and support are thus distributed across the entire lower quadrant of the breast with the left-to-right technique. The double Benelli advancement sutures have been used to bring the skin to the areola. As shown in the lateral view (Figure 12.8D), a normal contour has been restored and the fine "crumple lines" are fading on schedule.

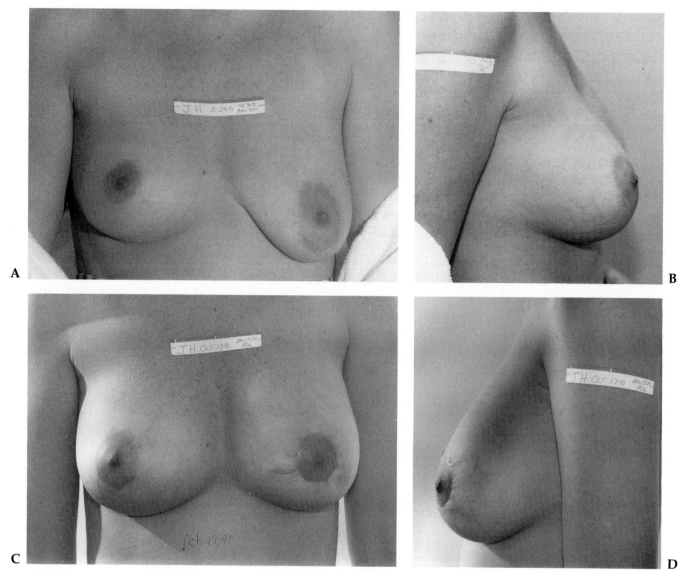

Figure 12.8. Case VIII: Bilateral breast augmentation and unilateral circumareolar mastopexy. See text for details.

Case IX: Areolar Expansion Following Secondary Augmentation of Circumareolar Reduction

A biopsy performed while the patient shown in Figure 12.9 was in Europe was shown to be malignant, and she flew home for definitive treatment (Figure 12.9A–C). She had complained about the size and weight of her breasts prior to this discovery. Our discussion centered on immediate reconstruction of the left breast; but with a normal mammogram and negative family history, the decision was made to do a circumareolar reduction on the right side. This would also help us to achieve a better balancing.

The procedures went well and the reconstruction was completed with a nipple graft as shown in Figure 12.9D. The circumareolar reduction maintained an excellent shape. However, 1 year later the patient decided to enlarge the breast on the right side as well as the left, and requested that a breast augmentation be performed.

As noted in Chapter 7 in this book, the problems of areolar expansion in the American series are of greater importance because many of the mastopexy patients also have breast augmentation prostheses placed at the same time. The weight and presence of a prosthesis plus the mechanical forces that it exerts were responsible for the stretching of the areola in the early series

and were likely responsible for some of the same problems in the modern era. This is illustrated by this patient (Figure 12.9E); 2 years following the augmentation of the right side, the areola has increased in diameter by almost a third. This expansion in February 1992 was left untreated until an unusual phenomenon occurred in November 1993, 3 years following reconstruction of the left breast. In a period of 1 month, this patient, and one other, both of whom had had breast reconstructions with polyurethane prosthesis, developed spontaneous hemorrhages! There was no history of trauma and no bruising was apparent. Our differential diagnosis included leishmaniasis, an infection caused by protozoans of the genus *Leishmania*, atypical mycobacteria *Staphylococcus epidermidis* infection, and spontaneous hemorrhage. All cultures, smears, and skin tests in both patients showed no evidence of bacteria and each has had an uneventful recovery after evacuation of the liquefied blood found within the polyurethane capsule. We are assuming that the weight of the polyurethane prosthesis created a mechanical problem leading to the hemorrhage shown in Figure 12.9F.

Each of the patients was explored within 24 hr and, in this case, having negative cultures and no evidence of infection, we proceeded to release the capsular contracture on the right and reduce the areola to a more acceptable shape.

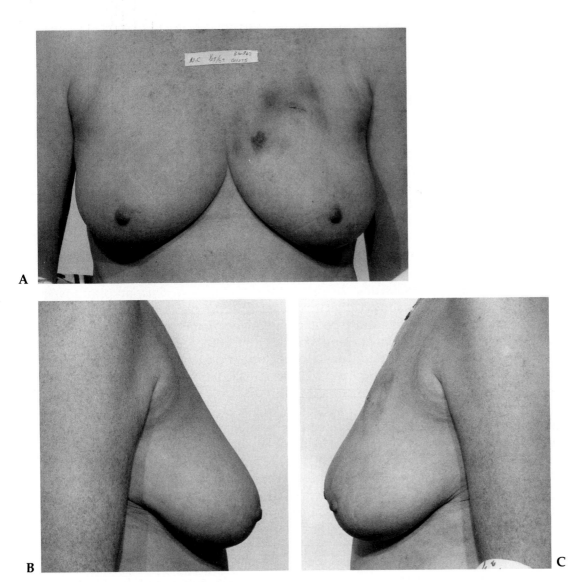

Figure 12.9. Case IX: Areolar expansion following secondary augmentation of circumareolar reduction. See text for details.

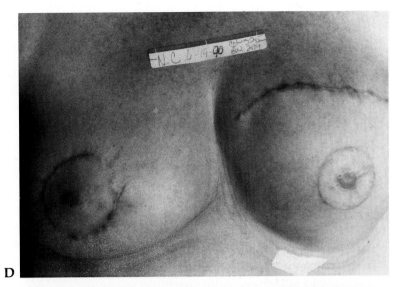

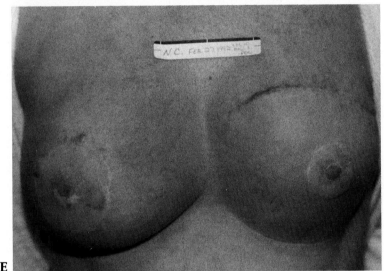

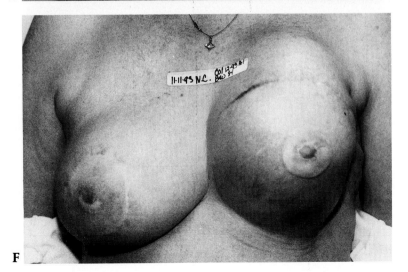

Case X

Figure 12.10 shows a patient 48 hr following implant removal and recreation of breasts by the circumareolar infolding technique. Mesh tape has been applied to stabilize the skin edges but the color of the areola on the right side has become dark.

The circumareolar technique is not immune to embarrassments of areolar circulation. In this case, removal of the first concentric suture restored color. A small hemorrhage, noted beneath the breast, was compressing the tissues. Nitroglycerin paste was not employed.

In the subsequent 48 hr nipple color returned to normal and sutures could be replaced without hazard. The patient has proceeded to an uneventful recovery.

Case XI: Moderate Reduction With Breast Prosthesis Removal

Typically, and fortunately, many patients who request implant removal do so because of the increased weight of the breasts, as illustrated by patient J.F. in Figure 12.11A. The additional soft tissue that has accumulated by weight gain or fibrocystic proliferation allows one to create a fuller, higher breast mound that is more suitable. Removing the prostheses accomplishes the aims of breast reduction: reducing bulk and weight. This patient illustrates the problem of areolar position made more difficult by the high position of the breast prosthesis shown in Figure 12.11A and B. The end result, seen from a lateral view (Figure 12.11C), is acceptable. However, the front view (Figure 12.11D) indicates that the areolae should have been set at least 2 cm higher. This would have given more tissue for infolding below to create a more conical mound than was achieved in this patient. It is important to understand that areolar upward migration does not occur with this type of repositioning and that one may proceed with an 18- or 19-cm position, as in ordinary breast reductions, without the fear of "star gazing."

References

1. Elliott MP: Mammoplasty for the tuberous breast. Ann Plast Surg 20:153, 1988.
2. Wilkinson T: Re: Elliott. Mammoplasty for the tuberous breast. Ann Plast Surg 21:294, 1988.

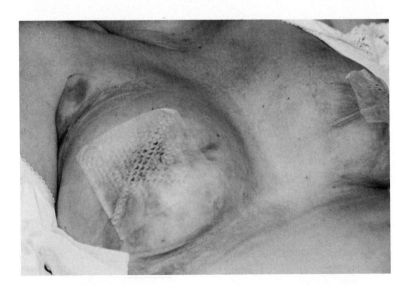

Figure 12.10. Case X: Embarrassment of areolar circulation.

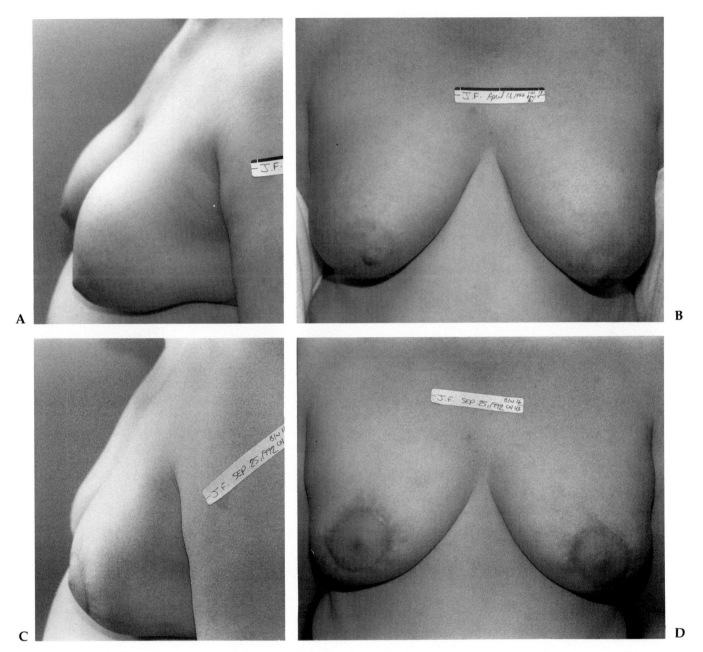

Figure 12.11. Case XI: Moderate reduction with breast prosthesis removal. See text for details.

Index